The Glucose Liberation

The 2-weeks Guide to Break free from the Cycle of Cravings,Boost your Metabolism and Reclaim Your Vitality

Jessica Luth

Copyright

Table of Content

Introduction

Thanks for coming to "The Glucose Liberation"! Do you get tired of feeling like your energy is going up and down like a roller coaster, leaving you feeling drained and defeated? When you give in to your cravings for sugary drinks and snacks, do you feel bad about yourself? Do you want to break out of the cycle of glucose imbalance and have a life full of energy, focus, and good health?

You're in the right place if so! This book will teach you about glucose, the amazing element that gives our bodies energy. This article will explain why glucose spikes are bad for you and how they can mess up your energy and digestion. You'll learn about the idea of trains, toasts, and Tetris, and how it can help you understand the impact of glucose imbalance on your body.

Don't worry, though; this book has more than just the problem. It also has the answer! We'll introduce you to the 2-Week Glucose Liberation Plan, a comprehensive program designed to help you reset and rebalance your glucose levels, and keep optimal energy and health. You'll learn how to feed your body tasty, healthy foods, how to work out to get more energy and speed up your metabolism, and how to deal with stress to keep your blood sugar levels in check.

Throughout this journey, we'll also provide you with a range of tools and resources to help you every step of the way. We'll give you everything you need to achieve, from meal plans and snack ideas to workout plans and ways to deal with stress.

So why wait? Join us on this trip to glucose liberation, and discover a life of boundless energy, clarity, and optimal health. Let's get started!

Chapter 1: Understanding Glucose

Caloric sweeteners come in a variety of forms and varieties, all of which are referred to as "sugar." Table sugar is the most widely known kind of sugar. Table sugar is technically defined as sucrose, a disaccharide composed of equal parts fructose and glucose, two monosaccharides.

Monosaccharides, sometimes known as "simple" sugars, are single units of sugar. We eat three main types of monosaccharides: glucose, galactose, and fructose. The three types of disaccharides (two connected sugar units) that are most significant for human nutrition are lactose, maltose, and sucrose. They combine in different combinations. The link between all of these is glucose. Maltose, which is made up of two linked glucose units, lactose, which is linked with galactose, and sucrose, which is linked with fructose, all contain it.

Not only is glucose essential to disaccharides, but it is also necessary for life. Our body uses glucose as its primary energy source, and certain tissues—like the brain—need a steady supply of it. Because it flows in our bloodstream as an immediately available energy source, glucose is known as "blood sugar." In addition, it is kept in the body as glycogen to be used as an energy source when the blood may not contain enough glucose.

From which does glucose originate?

The most prevalent monosaccharide in nature is glucose. It is produced by photosynthesis in plants. Certain plants use linked chains to store glucose. We refer to these chains as starch. Common foods that include starch include wheat, potatoes, corn, and rice. In order to produce dextrose, glucose, maltodextrins, polyols, and high fructose corn syrup, which are utilized as ingredients in the preparation of various foods, drinks, dressings, and sauces, starch is professionally separated from these complete food sources.

Several foods naturally contain glucose monosaccharides, however not as a component of starch. Honey is the most concentrated whole food source of glucose monosaccharides, followed by figs, dates, apricots, raisins, currants, cranberries, prunes, and dried fruits including dates and apricots.

Is glucose an added sugar or is it natural?

Depending on where it comes from, the sugar we eat is sometimes referred to as added sugar or natural sugar. When glucose is taken straight from whole foods like dates and apricots, it is regarded as a natural sugar. When taken from packaged goods and beverages that have had added glucose during production, it is regarded as an added sugar.

How does glucose break down?

It is not strictly necessary to metabolize glucose. Rather, it enters the bloodstream through the small intestine and is absorbed there, where it can either be used as an energy source or subsequently stored as glycogen in the liver and muscles.

In addition to obtaining glucose from foods and drinks that contain lactose, sucrose, and starch, we also directly take glucose from foods like honey. The saliva in our mouths must first convert starch into maltose, which are connected pairs of glucose units, when we eat foods high in starch. Following this, maltose is further broken down into its constituent glucose molecules, allowing for absorption. As with maltose digestion, glucose is absorbed from its companion monosaccharide (galactose in lactose and fructose in sucrose) only after it has been separated. When disaccharides and starches are broken down, glucose is absorbed more slowly and causes a smaller spike in blood sugar than when glucose is consumed directly.

Is it possible for our bodies to produce glucose?

For our bodies to work, glucose is necessary. Given that our brain consumes roughly 60% of the glucose that our bodies require, it is especially important for it. However, glucose does not necessarily need to be consumed right away from food and drink. The body produces glucose to make sure we always have enough of it. Breaking down glycogen to release the glucose it contains is one technique to accomplish this. Between meals or during moments of vigorous physical activity, glycogen is broken down. Gluconeogenesis is another method by which the body (mostly the liver) can create glucose from non-carbohydrate sources. When glucose intake is too low or nonexistent and glycogen stores are depleted, as happens during extended fasting or starvation, glucose synthesis takes place.

Chapter 2: Trains, Toasts, Tetris

Managing health can often feel like juggling multiple jobs at once. To simplify and understand the complex processes happening within our bodies, we can use relatable metaphors. Let's look into the metaphors of trains, toasts, and Tetris to gain a better picture of free radicals and oxidative stress, glycogen and inflammation, and insulin and fat gain.

Why the Trains Stop: Free Radicals and Oxidative Stress

Imagine your body as a vast network of train tracks, with trains representing different biological processes and functions. In an ideal situation, these trains run smoothly and efficiently, ensuring that everything from cell repair to nutrient delivery happens seamlessly. However, sometimes these trains come to a stop, causing delays and disruptions. This stoppage can be likened to the effect of free radicals and oxidative stress on your body.

What are Free Radicals?

Free radicals are unstable chemicals that contain an unpaired electron. They are natural results of metabolism but can also be introduced through external sources like pollution, radiation, and cigarette smoke. Because they are unstable, free radicals seek out other molecules to bond with, often harming cells, proteins, and DNA in the process.

Oxidative Stress

Oxidative stress happens when there is an imbalance between the production of free radicals and the body's ability to neutralize them with antioxidants. Antioxidants are molecules that can give an electron to a free radical without becoming destabilized themselves, thus neutralizing the threat.

The Consequences

When the "trains" stop due to oxidative stress, different adverse effects can occur:

1. Cellular Damage: Damaged cells can lead to a host of problems, including impaired performance and even cell death.

2. Accelerated Aging: Free radical damage is a big contributor to the aging process.

3. Chronic Diseases: Conditions such as cancer, cardiovascular diseases, and cognitive disorders have been linked to oxidative stress.

Managing Oxidative Stress

To keep your "trains" running smoothly, it's important to control oxidative stress:

1. Food: Consume a food rich in antioxidants. Foods like berries, nuts, green

leafy vegetables, and whole grains are great sources.

2. Lifestyle: Avoid smoking and excessive alcohol usage, and reduce exposure to environmental pollutants.

3. Supplements: In some cases, antioxidant supplements may be helpful, but it's best to consult with a healthcare provider.

Why Are You Toasting? Glycogen and Inflammation

Next, let's study the metaphor of toasting. Imagine your body's energy stores as slices of bread, and the process of converting these stores into useful energy as toasting the bread. When you eat carbohydrates, your body converts them into glucose, which is then stored as glycogen in your liver and muscles. This glycogen can be "toasted" or turned back into glucose when your body needs energy. However, just as over-toasting can burn the bread, improper control of glycogen can lead to inflammation.

Glycogen Storage and Usage

Glycogen is a form of stored glucose that serves as an easily available source of energy. When you need energy, such as during exercise or between meals, your body breaks down glycogen to keep blood glucose levels.

Inflammation

Inflammation is your body's natural reaction to injury or infection. However, chronic inflammation can result from poor glycogen management, leading to different health issues. When glycogen stores are consistently depleted and replenished in an unbalanced way, it can cause inflammatory responses.

The Role of Diet

Your diet plays a key role in managing glycogen levels and preventing inflammation:

1. Balanced Carbohydrate Intake: Ensure a balanced intake of carbohydrates to keep steady glycogen levels without causing spikes and crashes.

2. Healthy Fats: Incorporate healthy fats to support general metabolic health and reduce inflammation.

3. Antioxidants: Antioxidants also play a part in reducing inflammation by neutralizing free radicals.

Lifestyle Factors

In addition to diet, other lifestyle factors can affect glycogen and inflammation:

1. Regular Exercise: Physical exercise helps manage glycogen levels and reduce inflammation.

2. Adequate Rest: Ensure you get enough sleep and recovery time to support glycogen replenishment and general health.

Playing Tetris to Survive: Insulin and Fat Gain

Finally, let's look at the idea of playing Tetris. In the game of Tetris, you must fit various shapes into a confined area, much like your body must manage glucose and store excess as fat. Insulin is the hormone that facilitates this process, and when it functions optimally, it helps keep balance. However, if insulin levels are consistently high, it can lead to fat gain and other health problems.

Insulin and Glucose Management

Insulin is produced by the pancreas and helps cells to take in glucose from the bloodstream to use for energy or to store as fat. This process is important for maintaining stable blood sugar levels.

Insulin Resistance

When the body becomes resistant to insulin, it takes more insulin to manage blood sugar levels. This can lead to higher insulin levels in the blood, promoting fat storage, especially around the abdomen, and contributing to weight gain and metabolic disorders.

Factors Contributing to Insulin Resistance:

- Diet: Diets high in refined carbohydrates and sugars can lead to spikes in blood sugar and higher insulin production.

- Lack of Physical Activity: Sedentary lifestyles lead to poor glucose control and increased fat storage.

- Worry: Chronic worry can increase blood sugar levels and insulin resistance.

Understanding these metaphors—trains stopping for free radicals and oxidative stress, toasting for glycogen and inflammation, and playing Tetris for insulin and fat gain—can help simplify the complicated processes that affect your health. By recognizing these processes and implementing strategies to manage them, you can optimize your well-being and lower the chance of chronic diseases. Remember, it's about making informed choices and consistent efforts to support your body's natural processes, ensuring that your "trains" run smoothly, your "toast" is perfectly browned, and you become a master of your own metabolic "Tetris" game.

Chapter 3: The Impact of Glucose on Your Body and Mind

In our daily lives, we often hear about the importance of maintaining healthy blood sugar levels, but the depth of glucose's impact on our body and mind is seldom fully appreciated. Glucose, a simple sugar derived from the carbohydrates we eat, is essential for our survival. It fuels our cells, powers our muscles, and provides the necessary energy for our brain to function. However, when glucose levels are not properly managed, it can lead to a host of physical and mental health issues. Understanding how glucose affects your body and mind is crucial for making informed decisions about your diet and lifestyle.

The Physical Effects of Glucose

Glucose serves as a primary energy source for our body. When we consume carbohydrates, they are broken down into glucose, which enters the bloodstream. This process triggers the release of insulin, a hormone produced by the pancreas, which helps cells absorb glucose and use it for energy. This is a normal and healthy process, essential for our daily functioning. However, problems arise when glucose levels become too high or too low.

1. **High Blood Glucose Levels**

Persistently high blood glucose levels, a condition known as hyperglycemia, can have severe consequences. When there is too much glucose in the blood, it can lead to insulin resistance. Insulin resistance occurs when cells become less responsive to insulin, requiring more of the hormone to manage the same amount of glucose. Over time, this can lead to type 2 diabetes, a chronic condition characterized by high blood sugar levels and associated with numerous health complications, including heart disease, kidney damage, and vision problems.

High blood glucose levels also contribute to inflammation within the body. Chronic inflammation is linked to various conditions, including cardiovascular disease, cancer, and autoimmune disorders. Inflammation can damage blood vessels, leading to atherosclerosis (hardening of the arteries), which increases the risk of heart attacks and strokes.

2. Low Blood Glucose Levels

On the other hand, low blood glucose levels, or hypoglycemia, can also be dangerous. Hypoglycemia can occur when there is too much insulin in the bloodstream, often as a result of medications for diabetes, insufficient food intake, or excessive exercise. Symptoms of hypoglycemia include shakiness, sweating, confusion, irritability, and in severe cases, loss of consciousness or seizures. For individuals with diabetes, managing blood glucose levels is a constant balancing act to avoid both hyperglycemia and hypoglycemia.

3. Glucose and Energy Levels

Glucose directly impacts your energy levels. When your body efficiently uses glucose, you experience steady and sustained energy throughout the day. Conversely, poor glucose regulation can lead to energy highs and lows. Consuming foods high in refined sugars and simple carbohydrates causes rapid spikes in blood sugar, followed by sharp drops. These fluctuations can result in periods of high energy followed by crashes, leaving you feeling tired and lethargic.

Stable blood glucose levels are crucial for maintaining consistent energy. This can be achieved by consuming balanced meals that include complex carbohydrates, fiber, protein, and healthy fats. These components slow down the absorption of glucose, preventing rapid spikes and drops in blood sugar levels.

4. Cognitive Effects of Glucose

The brain, being one of the most glucose-demanding organs in the body, relies heavily on a steady supply of glucose to function optimally. This dependency makes the brain particularly sensitive to fluctuations in blood sugar levels.

5. Cognitive Function

Stable glucose levels are essential for cognitive function, including memory, attention, and decision-making. When blood glucose levels are too low, cognitive function can decline, leading to difficulties in concentration and impaired decision-making. This is because the brain lacks the necessary fuel to operate efficiently.

Conversely, chronic high blood glucose levels can negatively impact brain health. Studies have shown that prolonged hyperglycemia can lead to cognitive decline and increase the risk of neurodegenerative diseases such as Alzheimer's. High blood glucose levels can damage blood vessels in the brain, reducing blood flow and leading to brain cell damage.

6. Mood and Emotional Well-being

Glucose levels also have a significant impact on mood and emotional well-being. Fluctuations in blood sugar can affect neurotransmitter function, influencing mood regulation. For instance, low blood glucose levels can trigger the release of stress hormones like cortisol and adrenaline, leading to feelings of anxiety and irritability.

Moreover, the cycle of rapid glucose spikes and crashes associated with high sugar consumption can contribute to mood swings. This cycle can create a pattern of emotional highs and lows, where moments of elevated mood after sugar consumption are followed by crashes that leave you feeling down or depressed. Managing blood glucose levels through a balanced diet can help stabilize mood and improve emotional well-being.

Long-term Health Implications

The long-term health implications of poor glucose management are profound. Chronic high blood glucose levels are a significant risk factor for developing type 2 diabetes, a condition that affects millions of people worldwide. Diabetes is associated with severe complications, including cardiovascular disease, nerve damage, kidney failure, and vision loss.

Additionally, prolonged hyperglycemia can lead to insulin resistance, where the body requires increasing amounts of insulin to maintain normal blood sugar levels. This condition can progress to metabolic syndrome, a cluster of conditions that increase the risk of heart disease, stroke, and diabetes. Metabolic syndrome is characterized by high blood pressure, high blood sugar, excess body fat around the waist, and abnormal cholesterol levels.

Inflammation and Chronic Disease

Chronic inflammation, driven by persistently high blood glucose levels, is a key player in the development of many chronic diseases. Inflammation can damage tissues and organs over time, contributing to conditions such as cardiovascular disease, arthritis, and certain types of cancer. Managing glucose levels is crucial in reducing inflammation and lowering the risk of these chronic diseases.

Strategies for Managing Glucose Levels

Given the significant impact of glucose on your body and mind, managing blood glucose levels is essential for maintaining overall health and well-being. Here are some strategies to help you achieve stable glucose levels:

1. Balanced Diet:

Focus on a diet rich in whole foods, including fruits, vegetables, whole grains, lean proteins, and healthy fats. Avoid refined sugars and simple carbohydrates that cause rapid blood sugar spikes.

2. Regular Exercise:

Physical activity helps regulate blood glucose levels by increasing insulin sensitivity and promoting glucose uptake by muscles. Aim for a combination of aerobic exercise, strength training, and flexibility exercises.

3. **Mindful Eating:**

Pay attention to hunger and fullness cues, and avoid emotional eating. Eating mindfully can help prevent overeating and promote better glucose management.

4. **Consistent Meal Timing:**

Eating regular meals and snacks can help maintain steady blood sugar levels. Avoid skipping meals, which can lead to blood sugar fluctuations.

5. **Stress Management:**

Chronic stress can affect blood sugar levels. Incorporate stress-reducing practices such as meditation, yoga, deep breathing exercises, and adequate sleep into your daily routine.

6. **Hydration**:

Staying well-hydrated supports overall metabolic function and can help maintain stable blood glucose levels.

7. **Monitoring**:

If you have diabetes or are at risk, regularly monitoring your blood sugar levels can help you manage your condition more effectively. Work with your healthcare provider to develop a personalized plan.

The impact of glucose on your body and mind is profound and multifaceted. From fueling your cells and brain to influencing your mood and long-term health, glucose plays a critical role in your overall well-being. By understanding how glucose affects your body and implementing strategies to maintain stable blood sugar levels, you can improve your physical health, enhance cognitive function, and achieve a more balanced emotional state. Taking control of your glucose levels is a vital step towards a healthier, more vibrant life.

Chapter 4: Goals and Expectations for the Next Two Weeks

Embarking on a journey to improve your health and well-being is an empowering choice. Setting clear goals and expectations for the next two weeks is crucial for keeping focused, motivated, and on track.

Whether you're looking to break free from unhealthy habits, boost your metabolism, or reclaim your energy, having a roadmap to guide you along the way can make all the difference. Let's explore the goals and expectations you can set for yourself as you start on this transformative journey.

Clarifying Your Intentions

Before diving into detailed goals, take a moment to clarify your intentions for the next two weeks. What motivated you to start on this journey? What do you hope to achieve by the end of the two weeks? Whether it's improving your energy levels, losing weight, or simply feeling better in your body, knowing your underlying motivations will help you stay committed when faced with challenges.

Setting SMART Goals

When setting goals, it's important to make them SMART: Specific, Measurable, Achievable, Relevant, and Time-bound. This strategy ensures that your goals are clear, actionable, and realistic. Let's break down each component and apply it to your goals for the next two weeks.

Specific: Your goals should be clear and specific, leaving no room for doubt. Instead of saying, "I want to eat healthier," define what eating healthier means for you. For example, "I will incorporate at least two servings of vegetables into every meal."

Measurable: Your goals should be measurable so that you can track your progress and celebrate your successes. Include concrete metrics or milestones to gauge your progress. For instance, "I will aim to drink eight glasses of water per day."

Achievable: While it's important to challenge yourself, your goals should also be realistic and achievable within the given timeframe. Consider your present lifestyle, commitments, and resources when setting goals. For example, if you're new to exercise, committing to an hour of intense workouts every day may not be possible. Start with smaller, more attainable goals and gradually increase the intensity as you grow.

Relevant: Your goals should align with your overarching aims and be relevant to your health and well-being. Focus on goals that will have a meaningful effect on your life and contribute to your overall well-being. For example, if your goal is to improve your sleep quality, making a goal to reduce screen time before bed would be relevant and beneficial.

Time-bound: Give yourself a deadline to work towards, which provides a sense of urgency and accountability. Setting a time-bound goal ensures that you stay focused and inspired to take action. For example, "I will meditate for 10 minutes every morning before starting my day."

Example Goals for the Next Two Weeks

Now that we've established the SMART criteria for setting goals, let's describe some example goals you can set for yourself over the next two weeks. Remember to tailor these goals to your individual wants, preferences, and circumstances.

1. **Nutrition Goals:**

Specific: Incorporate a range of fruits and vegetables into every meal.

Measurable: Aim for at least five servings of fruits and veggies per day.

Achievable: Start by adding one extra serving of fruits or vegetables to each meal and gradually increase as you feel safe.

Relevant: Improving your diet by increasing fruit and vegetable intake can provide important vitamins, minerals, and antioxidants, supporting overall health.

Time-bound: Commit to this goal for the next two weeks and track your progress daily.

2. **Physical Activity Goals:**

Specific: Establish a consistent exercise routine that includes a mix of cardiovascular exercise, strength training, and flexibility exercises.

Measurable: Aim for at least 30 minutes of moderate-intensity exercise on most days of the week.

Achievable: Start with shorter workout sessions and gradually increase length and intensity as your fitness improves.

Relevant: Regular physical exercise has numerous health benefits, including improved cardiovascular health, increased energy levels, and enhanced mood.

Time-bound: Commit to exercising at least five days a week for the next two weeks and track your workouts to monitor growth.

3. Stress Management Goals:

Specific: Incorporate daily stress-relief techniques, such as meditation, deep breathing exercises, or spending time in nature.

Measurable: Dedicate at least 10 minutes each day to stress-relief tasks.

Achievable: Start with short, manageable sessions and gradually increase length as you become more comfortable.

Relevant: Managing stress is important for overall well-being and can help improve sleep quality, reduce anxiety, and enhance resilience.

Time-bound: Commit to practicing stress-relief techniques everyday for the next two weeks and track your progress.

3. Hydration Goals:

Specific: Increase water intake to ensure proper hydration throughout the day.

Measurable: Aim to drink at least eight glasses (64 ounces) of water per day.

Achievable: Carry a reusable water bottle with you throughout the day as a reminder to drink regularly.

Relevant: Staying hydrated is important for maintaining proper bodily processes, supporting digestion, circulation, and temperature regulation.

Time-bound: Commit to meeting your daily hydration goal for the next two weeks and track your water intake using a hydration app or journal.

Managing Expectations

While setting goals is essential for success, it's equally important to manage your expectations and be flexible with your approach. Understand that growth is not always linear, and there may be obstacles or setbacks along the way. Be patient with yourself and celebrate small wins, no matter how insignificant they may seem.

Additionally, remember that making lasting change takes time and consistency. The habits you create over the next two weeks are the building blocks for long-term health and well-being. Focus on making sustainable living changes rather than quick fixes or short-term solutions.

Week 1: Breaking Free from Cravings

Day1: Recognizing and Understanding Cravings

Welcome to Day 1 of your journey to break free from cravings. Today, we will dig into the science behind cravings and identify common triggers. Understanding these factors is crucial as it lays the foundation for overcoming them and developing healthier habits.

The Science Behind Cravings

Cravings are powerful and often sudden urges to eat specific foods, usually high in sugar, salt, or fat. Unlike hunger, which is a natural need for food, cravings are driven by the brain and can occur even when we are not physically hungry. To successfully manage cravings, it's important to understand the underlying mechanisms that trigger them.

The Brain's Reward System

At the core of cravings lies the brain's reward system, which is designed to reinforce behaviors that are important for survival, such as eating. When we eat food, especially those high in sugar and fat, our brain releases dopamine, a neurotransmitter associated with pleasure and reward. This release provides a pleasurable sensation, encouraging us to repeat the action. Over time, our brains can become conditioned to seek out these foods to experience the same pleasurable reaction, leading to cravings.

Hormonal Influences

Hormones also play a major role in cravings. Two key hormones involved are ghrelin and leptin. Ghrelin, often referred to as the "hunger hormone," tells your brain that it's time to eat. When ghrelin levels are high, you may feel increased appetite and cravings. On the other hand, leptin, known as the "satiety hormone," tells your brain when you are full. Imbalances in these hormones can disrupt regular hunger signals, leading to overeating and cravings.

Blood Sugar Levels

Fluctuations in blood sugar levels can trigger cravings, especially for sugary and high-carb foods. When you consume refined sugars and simple carbohydrates, they are quickly absorbed into the bloodstream, causing a spike in blood sugar levels.

In reaction, your body releases insulin to help cells absorb the glucose. This rapid spike is often followed by a sharp drop in blood sugar levels, leading to feelings of fatigue and a renewed desire for more sugar to boost energy levels.

Emotional and Psychological Factors

Cravings are not solely driven by physiological factors; emotional and psychological aspects play a major role as well. Stress, anxiety, boredom, and other emotions can trigger cravings as a form of coping strategy. For many, food provides comfort and briefly alleviates negative emotions. This emotional eating can become a habitual reaction, reinforcing the cycle of cravings.

Common Triggers

Recognizing the common triggers that lead to cravings is the first step towards controlling them effectively. By identifying these triggers, you can create strategies to handle and mitigate them. Here are some of the most popular triggers:

1. **Stress**

Stress is a significant trigger for cravings, especially for high-sugar and high-fat foods. When you're worried, your body releases cortisol, a hormone that increases appetite and can lead to cravings for comfort foods. Finding healthy ways to handle stress, such as exercise, meditation, or deep breathing exercises, can help reduce stress-induced cravings.

2. **Lack of Sleep**

Sleep deprivation affects the balance of hunger-regulating hormones, increasing levels of ghrelin and lowering levels of leptin. This hormonal imbalance can lead to increased appetite and cravings, especially for calorie-dense foods. Prioritizing good sleep hygiene and looking for 7-9 hours of sleep per night can help regulate these hormones and reduce cravings.

3. Dehydration

Sometimes, hunger can be a sign of dehydration. When your body is dehydrated, it can send cues that are similar to hunger, leading you to eat when you really just need to drink water. Ensuring that you stay adequately hydrated throughout the day can help distinguish between real hunger and dehydration-related cravings.

4. **Nutrient Deficiencies**

Cravings can also be a sign that your body is missing certain nutrients. For example, a desire for chocolate might indicate a magnesium deficiency, while a craving for salty foods could be a sign of low sodium levels. Eating a balanced meal rich in a variety of nutrients can help address these deficiencies and reduce cravings.

5. **Habitual and Environmental Cues**

Certain habits and environmental cues can cause cravings. For instance, if you always eat a snack while watching TV, the act of sitting down to watch your favorite show may trigger a desire for a snack, even if you're not hungry. Similarly, seeing ads for food or walking past a bakery can trigger cravings. Becoming aware of these cues can help you create strategies to break these associations.

6. Emotional Triggers

Emotions like sadness, loneliness, and boredom can drive cravings for comfort foods. Identifying emotional triggers and finding alternative ways to deal with these feelings, such as talking to a friend, engaging in a hobby, or practicing mindfulness, can help reduce emotional eating.

7. Social Influences

Social settings, such as gatherings with friends or family, can also trigger cravings. Being around others who are indulging in tempting foods can make it difficult to avoid cravings. Planning ahead and finding ways to enjoy social settings without giving in to unhealthy cravings can help you stay on track.

Strategies for Managing Cravings

Now that you understand the science behind cravings and common triggers, let's explore some strategies to handle them effectively.

1. Eat Balanced Meals

Consuming balanced meals that include protein, healthy fats, and carbs can help keep blood sugar levels stable and reduce cravings. These nutrients help slow the absorption of glucose into the bloodstream, avoiding rapid spikes and drops in blood sugar levels.

2. Practice Mindful Eating

Mindful eating involves paying attention to what and how you eat, enjoying each bite, and listening to your body's hunger and fullness cues. By eating carefully, you can better distinguish between true hunger and cravings, and make more intentional food choices.

3. Manage Stress

Incorporate stress-management methods into your daily routine, such as exercise, meditation, deep breathing exercises, or engaging in hobbies. Reducing stress can help lower cortisol levels and lessen stress-induced cravings.

4. Stay Hydrated

Drink plenty of water throughout the day to stay refreshed. Sometimes, thirst can be mistaken for hunger, leading to needless eating. Keeping a water bottle with you and drinking regularly can help avoid dehydration-related cravings.

5. Get Adequate Sleep

Prioritize good sleep hygiene and try for 7-9 hours of sleep per night. Consistent, quality sleep helps control hunger hormones and can reduce cravings. Establish a regular sleep schedule and build a relaxing bedtime routine to improve sleep quality.

6. Plan and Prepare Healthy Snacks

Having healthy snacks readily available can help you make better choices when cravings hit. Prepare a variety of nutritious snacks, such as cut-up vegetables, nuts, yogurt, or fruit, so you have healthy choices on hand.

7. Identify and Address Emotional Triggers

Reflect on your emotional triggers and find alternative ways to deal with negative emotions. Engaging in activities that bring you joy, talking to a friend, or practicing mindfulness can help you handle emotional triggers without turning to food.

8. Create a Supportive Environment

Surround yourself with supportive people and build an environment that promotes healthy choices. Remove unhealthy temptations from your home and stock your kitchen with nutritious foods. Having a support system can help you stay accountable and inspired. Recognizing and knowing cravings is the first step in breaking free from their hold. By understanding the science behind cravings and identifying common triggers, you can develop effective strategies to control them.

Today, take some time to think on your own cravings and the triggers that may be influencing them. With this knowledge, you can begin to make mindful choices that support your journey towards better health and well-being. Remember, this is just the beginning, and each step you take brings you closer to breaking free from cravings and meeting your health goals.

Day 2: Clean Out Your Pantry

Welcome to Day 2 of your journey to break free from cravings and recover your vitality. Today, we focus on changing your pantry. Cleaning out your pantry is a crucial step in setting yourself up for success. By eliminating temptations and stocking up on healthy alternatives, you create an atmosphere that supports your goals and makes healthier choices more approachable.

The Importance of a Healthy Pantry

Your pantry is the heart of your kitchen, and its contents can significantly affect your eating habits. When your pantry is stocked with nutritious options, making healthy choices becomes easy. Conversely, a pantry filled with sugary snacks, processed foods, and unhealthy pleasures can derail your efforts. Taking the time to clean out and restock your pantry sets the stage for long-term success and helps you stay on track with your health goals.

Eliminating Temptations

The first step in cleaning out your pantry is to remove temptations. These are the foods that spark cravings and make it difficult to stick to a healthy eating plan. Here's a step-by-step guide to help you clean and detoxify your pantry:

1. Take Inventory

Start by taking a thorough inventory of your pantry. Pull out all the things and lay them on your kitchen counter. This allows you to see everything you have and rate each item individually. Be honest with yourself about which foods are helpful and which are harmful to your goals.

2. **Identify Unhealthy Foods**

Identify foods that do not align with your health goals. Common causes include:

- Sugary Snacks: Cookies, candy, chocolate bars, and cakes.
- Processed Foods: Chips, snacks, instant noodles, and microwave meals.
- Sugary Beverages: Sodas, sugary juices, and energy drinks.
- Refined Carbohydrates: White bread, white rice, and sugary sweets.
- High-Fat and High-Sodium Foods: Packaged snack foods, processed meats, and fast food items.

These foods are often high in sugar, unhealthy fats, and empty calories. They provide little nutritional value and can cause cravings, making it harder to stick to your health plan.

3. **Discard or Donate**

Once you've discovered the unhealthy foods, decide what to do with them. If an item is unopened and non-perishable, consider giving it to a local food bank or shelter. For opened or perishable things, it's best to discard them. This step may feel unnecessary, but think of it as an investment in your health. Removing these temptations from your surroundings is a powerful step towards achieving your goals.

4. **Clean and Organize**

After removing unhealthy items, take the chance to clean and organize your pantry. Wipe down shelves, vacuum any crumbs, and ensure everything is clean. A clean and organized pantry makes it easier to see what you have and quickly access healthy choices.

Stocking Up on Healthy Alternatives

With the temptations removed, it's time to restock your pantry with nutritious, wholesome foods. Here's how to ensure your pantry is filled with healthy choices that support your journey:

1. **Whole Grains and Complex Carbohydrates**

Whole grains and complex carbohydrates provide sustained energy and are rich in fiber, which helps keep you full and happy. Some excellent choices include:

- Quinoa
- Brown Rice
- Oats
- Whole Wheat Pasta
- Barley

These grains can be the basis of many healthy meals and are versatile enough to be used in various recipes.

2. **Protein Sources**

Protein is important for muscle repair, immune function, and maintaining satiety. Stock up on a range of protein sources, such as:

- Canned Beans: Black beans, chickpeas, and lentils.
- Nuts and Seeds: Almonds, walnuts, chia seeds, and flaxseeds.
- Nut Butters: Almond butter, peanut butter (look for natural choices without added sugars or hydrogenated oils).
- Canned Fish: Tuna, salmon, and sardines (opt for forms packed in water or olive oil).

These protein sources are convenient, versatile, and can be incorporated into different meals and snacks.

3. Healthy Fats

Healthy fats are important for brain function, hormone production, and overall health. Include a range of healthy fats in your pantry, such as:

- Olive Oil: Use for cooking, salad sauces, and marinades.
- Avocado Oil: Great for high-heat cooking.
- Coconut Oil: Versatile for both cooking and baking.
- Nuts and Seeds: In addition to being protein sources, they are also rich in healthy fats.

Incorporating these fats into your diet can help you feel more full and less likely to crave unhealthy foods.

4. Snacks and Treats

It's important to have healthy snacks and treats available to curb cravings without derailing your diet. Some nutritious snack choices include:

- Fresh Fruit: Apples, oranges, berries, and citrus fruits.
- Dried Fruit: Look for options without extra sugars, such as dried apricots, figs, and dates.
- Dark Chocolate: Choose chocolate with at least 70% cocoa content for a healthy treat.
- Popcorn: Air-popped popcorn is a low-calorie, high-fiber snack.

These snacks can provide a quick energy boost and fill your sweet or savory cravings in a healthier way.

5. Herbs, Spices, and Flavorings

Enhancing the taste of your meals with herbs and spices can make healthy eating more enjoyable and satisfying. Stock your pantry with a range of seasonings, such as:

- Spices: Cinnamon, ginger, cumin, paprika, and black pepper.
- Herbs: Dried basil, oregano, thyme, rosemary, and parsley.
- Flavorings: Garlic powder, onion powder, and chili flakes.

Experimenting with different herbs and spices can add excitement to your meals and help you discover new flavor combinations.

6. Condiments and Add-Ins

Choose healthier condiments and add-ins that improve your meals without adding excessive sugar, salt, or unhealthy fats. Some choices include:

- Mustard
- Balsamic Vinegar
- Hot Sauce
- Tamari or Low-Sodium Soy Sauce
- Nutritional Yeast

These things can be used to add flavor to your dishes without compromising your health goals.

Creating a Meal Plan

With your pantry stocked with healthy alternatives, it's time to create a meal plan that uses these nutritious ingredients. Planning your meals in advance helps you stay organized, reduces the desire to order takeout, and ensures you're consuming a balanced diet. Here are some tips for successful meal planning:

1. Plan Balanced Meals

Ensure that each meal includes a mix of protein, healthy fats, complex carbohydrates, and vegetables. This combination helps keep you full and satisfied, reducing the chance of cravings.

2. Prepare Snacks in Advance

Having healthy snacks readily available can prevent you from reaching for unhealthy options when hunger hits. Pre-portion snacks like nuts, seeds, fruit, and veggies into individual servings for ease.

3. Batch Cooking

Consider batch cooking meals and freezing parts for later use. This saves time during busy days and ensures you always have a healthy option open. Some batch-cooking ideas include soups, stews, casseroles, and grain bowls.

4. **Incorporate Variety**

To avoid boredom and ensure you're getting a range of nutrients, incorporate variety into your meal plan. Try different grains, proteins, and veggies each week, and play with new recipes and flavor combinations.

5. **Stay Flexible**

While planning is important, it's also necessary to stay flexible. Life can be uncertain, and there may be days when your planned meals don't go as expected. Keep some quick and easy meal options on hand, such as canned beans, frozen veggies, and whole grain pasta, to help you stay on track.

Cleaning out your pantry and restocking it with healthy choices is a powerful step towards breaking free from cravings and achieving your health goals. By eliminating temptations and building a supportive environment, you set yourself up for success.

Remember, the goal is not to deprive yourself but to make healthier choices more approachable and enjoyable. With a well-stocked pantry and a strong meal plan, you are well on your way to a healthier, more vibrant you. Stay committed, stay motivated, and accept the positive changes you're making in your life.

Day 3: The Power of Balanced Meals

Welcome to Day 3 of your journey towards breaking free from cravings and reclaiming your energy. Today, we will explore the power of balanced meals and the important role macronutrients play in your diet. Understanding macronutrients and how to incorporate them into your meals can help you maintain energy levels, support overall health, and avoid cravings. We'll also provide sample meal plans to guide you in making balanced, nutritious meals.

Macronutrients Explained

Macronutrients are the nutrients your body needs in large amounts to function properly. They include carbs, proteins, and fats. Each macronutrient plays a unique and important role in your body's health and performance.

1. Carbohydrates

Carbohydrates are the body's main source of energy. They are broken down into glucose, which feeds your brain, muscles, and other tissues. There are two main types of carbohydrates: simple and complicated.

Simple Carbohydrates: These are quickly digested and can cause fast spikes in blood sugar levels. They include sugars found in fruits, milk, and honey, as well as refined sugars in sweets, drinks, and baked goods.

Complex Carbohydrates: These are digested more slowly and provide a steady flow of energy. They include whole grains, legumes, veggies, and fruits.

Benefits of Carbohydrates:

- Provide energy for physical exercise and brain function.

- Supply fiber, which helps digestion and promotes satiety.

- Include important vitamins and minerals.

2. Proteins

Proteins are the building blocks of your body. They are made up of amino acids, which are necessary for the growth, repair, and maintenance of tissues. There are complete proteins (containing all essential amino acids) and incomplete proteins (lacking one or more necessary amino acids).

- **Complete Proteins**: Found in animal goods like meat, fish, poultry, eggs, and dairy.

-**Incomplete Proteins:** Found in plant-based foods like beans, lentils, nuts, seeds, and whole grains.

Benefits of Proteins:

- Support muscle growth and repair.

- Boost the defense system.

- Help in the production of enzymes and hormones.

- Aid in keeping healthy skin, hair, and nails.

3. Fats

Fats are important for various bodily functions, including energy storage, nutrient absorption, and hormone production. There are different types of fats: unsaturated, saturated, and trans fats.

- **Unsaturated Fats**: Considered good fats, found in olive oil, avocados, nuts, seeds, and fatty fish.
- **Saturated Fats:** Found in animal goods like meat and dairy, as well as tropical oils like coconut oil. These should be taken in moderation.
- **Trans Fats**: Found in many processed foods and should be avoided as they can increase the risk of heart disease.

Benefits of Fats:

- Provide a strong source of energy.

- Support cell growth and protect organs.

- Aid in the absorption of fat-soluble vitamins (A, D, E, and K).

- Promote brain health and hormonal balance.

The Importance of Balanced Meals

A balanced meal includes a healthy proportion of carbohydrates, proteins, and fats, along with vitamins, minerals, and fiber. Eating balanced meals helps control blood sugar levels, maintain energy throughout the day, and keep you feeling full and satisfied. Here's how you can make balanced meals:

1. **Portion Control**

Balance the amounts of macronutrients on your plate. A general guideline is to fill half of your plate with veggies and fruits, a quarter with lean protein, and a quarter with whole grains or starchy vegetables. Include a small amount of healthy fats to improve flavor and satiety.

2. **Variety**

Incorporate a range of foods from each macronutrient group. Different foods provide different nutrients, so eating a wide range of foods ensures you get all the important nutrients your body needs.

3. **Nutrient Density**

Choose nutrient-dense foods that provide more vitamins, minerals, and fiber compared to their calorie content. Focus on whole, unprocessed foods like veggies, fruits, whole grains, lean proteins, and healthy fats.

4. Timing

Eat regular meals and snacks throughout the day to keep energy levels and prevent overeating. Skipping meals can lead to cravings and bad food choices later in the day.

Sample Meal Plans

To help you get started with healthy meals, here are some sample meal plans for breakfast, lunch, and dinner. These plans include a mix of macronutrients and nutrient-dense foods to keep you energized and pleased.

Breakfast

1. Oatmeal with Berries and Nuts
   - 1 cup of cooked oatmeal
   - 1/2 cup of mixed berries (strawberries, blueberries, raspberries)
   - 1 tablespoon of chopped nuts (almonds, walnuts, or pecans)
   - 1 teaspoon of chia seeds

- A drop of honey or maple syrup (optional)
- A splash of milk or a dairy-free option

Benefits: This breakfast offers complex carbohydrates from oats, antioxidants and vitamins from berries, healthy fats and protein from nuts and chia seeds, and a touch of sweetness without refined sugars.

2. Greek Yogurt Parfait

- 1 cup of Greek yogurt (plain or low-fat)
- 1/2 cup of granola (look for low-sugar choices)
- 1/2 cup of fresh fruit (banana slices, berries, or kiwi)
- 1 tablespoon of flaxseeds or hemp seeds

Benefits: Greek yogurt is a great source of protein, granola adds fiber and crunch, and fresh fruit offers vitamins and natural sweetness. Seeds add extra nutrients and good fats.

Lunch

1. Quinoa Salad with Grilled Chicken
   - 1 cup of cooked quinoa
   - 1 grilled chicken breast, sliced
   - 1 cup of mixed greens (spinach, arugula, or kale)
   - 1/2 cup of cherry tomatoes, halved - 1/4 cup of cucumber, diced
   - 1/4 cup of feta cheese, crumbled
   - A handful of olives
   - Olive oil and lemon juice dressing

Benefits: This salad is a perfect mix of protein, fiber, healthy fats, and complex carbohydrates. The veggies provide vitamins and antioxidants, while the dressing adds flavor and healthy fats.

2. Lentil Soup with Whole Grain Bread

- 1 cup of cooked lentils
- 1 cup of vegetable broth
- 1/2 cup of diced carrots
- 1/2 cup of diced celery
- 1/2 cup of diced tomatoes
- 1/4 cup of chopped onion
- 2 cloves of garlic, minced
- 1 tablespoon of olive oil
- Herbs and spices (thyme, bay leaf, salt, and pepper)
- 1 slice of whole grain bread

Benefits: Lentils are a great source of plant-based energy and fiber. The vegetables add vitamins and minerals, while the whole grain bread offers complex carbohydrates to keep you full.

Dinner

1. **Baked Salmon with Roasted Vegetables**
   - 1 salmon fillet
   - 1 cup of mixed veggies (broccoli, bell peppers, and zucchini)
   - 1 tablespoon of olive oil
   - Herbs and spices (dill, garlic powder, lemon juice, salt, and pepper)
   - 1/2 cup of brown rice or quinoa

Benefits: Salmon is rich in omega-3 fatty acids, which are helpful for heart and brain health. The roasted veggies provide fiber and nutrients, while the brown rice or quinoa adds complex carbohydrates.

2. Chicken Stir-Fry with Brown Rice

- 1 chicken breast, sliced
- 1 cup of mixed veggies (bell peppers, snap peas, carrots, and broccoli)
- 1/2 cup of brown rice
- 1 tablespoon of olive oil or sesame oil
- 2 cloves of garlic, chopped
- 1 tablespoon of low-sodium soy sauce or tamari
- 1 teaspoon of ginger, grated

Benefits: This stir-fry is a balanced meal with lean protein, fiber-rich veggies, and complex carbohydrates. The garlic and ginger add flavor and anti-inflammatory qualities.

Creating balanced meals with the right mix of macronutrients is important for keeping energy levels, supporting overall health, and preventing cravings. By knowing the roles of carbohydrates, proteins, and fats, you can make informed choices about the foods you eat. The sample meal plans given can serve as a guide to help you get started on your journey to healthier eating. Remember, the key to success is variety, amount control, and nutrient density. With these ideas in mind, you are well on your way to achieving your health and wellness goals. Keep up the great work and enjoy the good changes you are making in your life.

Day 4: Mindful Eating

Welcome to Day 4 of your journey to break free from cravings, improve your metabolism, and reclaim your vitality. Today, we will focus on mindful eating, a practice that pushes you to be present and fully engaged during your meals. Mindful eating can help you build a healthier relationship with food, improve digestion, and prevent overeating. By incorporating mindfulness methods and understanding their benefits, you can make more conscious, satisfying food choices.

Mindful eating is about paying attention to your food and the experience of eating without distraction. It includes acknowledging your hunger and satiety cues, savoring each bite, and recognizing the effects of food on your body and mind. This exercise can transform your eating habits and help you appreciate food as nourishment rather than just fuel.

Techniques for Mindfulness

1. Set an Intention

Before you begin your meal, set a goal for mindful eating. This can be as easy as deciding to eat slowly, savor each bite, or listen to your body's hunger and fullness signals. Setting an intention helps you focus on the present time and enhances your awareness.

2. Eliminate Distractions

Create a calm and distraction-free setting for eating. Turn off the television, put away your phone, and sit down at a table. Eliminating distractions helps you to fully engage with your meal and the experience of eating.

3. Engage Your Senses

Pay attention to the colors, textures, and smells of your food. Notice how it looks on your plate, how it smells, and how it feels in your mouth. Engaging your senses helps you connect with your food on a deeper level and improves the pleasure of eating.

4. Chew Thoroughly

Chew your food slowly and carefully. This not only aids digestion but also allows you to enjoy the flavors and textures of each bite. Aim to chew each bite 20-30 times before swallowing. Chewing fully can also help you feel fuller faster, preventing overeating.

5. Pause Between Bites

Put your fork down between bites and take a moment to breathe. Pausing between bites gives your body time to register fullness and stops you from eating too quickly. It also lets you to enjoy the conversation if you're dining with others.

6. Listen to Your Body

Pay attention to your body's hunger and fullness cues. Eat when you're hungry, and stop when you're comfortably full. Mindful eating encourages you to respect your body's signals rather than external cues, such as the time of day or the amount of food on your plate.

7. Reflect on Your Meal

After eating, take a moment to think on your meal. How did the food taste? How do you feel physically and emotionally? Reflecting on your meal helps you build a positive relationship with food and understand how different foods affect your well-being.

Benefits of Mindful Eating

Practicing thoughtful eating offers numerous benefits for both your physical and mental health. Here are some of the key advantages:

1. Improved Digestion

Eating mindfully and chewing thoroughly can improve digestion. When you eat slowly and chew your food well, you break down food bits more effectively, making it easier for your digestive system to process nutrients. This can lead to decreased bloating, gas, and digestive discomfort.

2. Better Nutrient Absorption

Mindful eating can improve nutrient absorption by helping your body to process food more effectively. When you eat slowly and mindfully, your body has more time to make digestive enzymes and absorb nutrients from the food you consume.

3. Enhanced Satisfaction and Enjoyment

Focusing on the sensory experience of eating can improve your enjoyment and satisfaction with your meals. By savoring each bite and appreciating the flavors, textures, and aromas of your food, you can receive more pleasure from eating.

4. Reduced Overeating

Mindful eating helps you notice your body's hunger and fullness cues, preventing overeating. By listening to your body and eating only when you're hungry, you can avoid consuming excess calories and lower the risk of weight gain.

5. Improved Relationship with Food

Mindful eating fosters a healthier relationship with food by promoting awareness and appreciation. It helps you move away from emotional eating and recognize food as nourishment rather than a coping strategy for stress or boredom.

6. Stress Reduction

Practicing mindfulness during meals can lower stress and promote relaxation. Eating in a calm and focused way activates the parasympathetic nervous system, which helps counteract the stress response and supports overall well-being.

7. Increased Awareness of Eating Patterns

Mindful eating can help you become more aware of your eating trends and habits. By paying attention to what, when, and how much you eat, you can identify triggers for unhealthy eating habits and make more conscious choices.

Mindful eating is a powerful practice that can transform your relationship with food and support your general health and well-being. By incorporating mindfulness methods and understanding the benefits, you can make more conscious, satisfying food choices. Start by setting a goal for mindful eating, eliminating distractions, engaging your senses, and listening to your body's cues. With practice, mindful eating can become a natural and fun part of your daily routine, helping you achieve your health goals and enjoy a more balanced, nourishing life.

Day 5: Healthy Snacking Strategies

Welcome to Day 5 of your two-week journey toward breaking free from cravings, boosting your metabolism, and reclaiming your energy. Today, we will focus on healthy snacking tactics. Snacking often gets a bad rap, but when done thoughtfully, it can play a crucial role in maintaining your energy levels, stabilizing blood sugar, and supporting general health. We'll explore smart snacking choices and provide some delicious and healthy recipe ideas to help you make the most of your snacks.

Smart Snacking Choices

The key to healthy snacking is choosing nutrient-dense foods that provide sustained energy and important nutrients without causing blood sugar spikes or excessive calorie intake. Here are some tips to help you make smart eating choices:

1. Focus on Nutrient Density

Opt for snacks that are rich in vitamins, minerals, fiber, and protein. Nutrient-dense snacks provide more nutritional value per calorie, helping you stay fuller for longer and avoid empty calories found in many processed snacks.

Examples:
- Fresh fruits and veggies
- Nuts and seeds
- Whole carbs
- Low-fat dairy or dairy alternatives
- Lean foods

2. Combine Macronutrients

Macronutrients—carbohydrates, proteins, and fats—can help make a balanced snack that keeps you satisfied. Carbohydrates provide quick energy, proteins help build and repair tissues, and fats are important for brain health and satiety.

Examples:
- Apple pieces with almond butter
- Greek yogurt with berries and chia seeds
- Whole grain crackers with cheese
- Hummus with carrot sticks

3. Watch Portion Sizes

Even healthy snacks can lead to overeating if not portioned properly. Be mindful of serving sizes to avoid taking too many calories. Pre-portion your snacks at the beginning of the week to make it easy to grab a healthy portion on the go.

Examples:

- A small handful of nuts (about 1 ounce)
- A single-serving jar of Greek yogurt
- A few pieces of dark chocolate (about 1 ounce)
- A small bowl of air-popped popcorn (about 3 cups)

4. Avoid Added Sugars and Unhealthy Fats

Many packaged snacks contain extra sugars, unhealthy fats, and artificial chemicals. Reading labels and picking whole, unprocessed foods can help you avoid these pitfalls and make healthier choices.

Examples:

- Opt for plain yogurt and sweeten it with fresh fruit instead of sweetened yogurts with added sugars.

- Choose whole fruits instead of fruit snacks or candies.

- Make your own trail mix with nuts, seeds, and dried fruit, avoiding pre-packaged mixes with added sugars and oils.

5. Stay Hydrated

Sometimes what feels like hunger is actually thirst. Staying hydrated can help avoid unnecessary snacking and support overall health. Drink water throughout the day and consider incorporating hydrating snacks like fruits and veggies with high water content.

Examples:
- Cucumber slices with a splash of lemon juice
- Watermelon bits
- Celery sticks with hummus - A drink made with water or coconut water as the base

Recipe Ideas

Here are some healthy, easy-to-make snack ideas that are both delicious and nutritious. These recipes combine a balance of macronutrients and nutrient-dense ingredients to keep you satisfied between meals.

1. Energy Balls

Energy balls are a great grab-and-go snack that combines healthy fats, proteins, and carbohydrates. They're easy to make and can be customized with your favorite seasonings.

Ingredients:

- 1 cup rolled oats

- 1/2 cup nut butter (almond, peanut, or cashew)

- 1/4 cup honey or maple syrup

- 1/4 cup flaxseeds or chia seeds

- 1/4 cup dark chocolate chips or dried fruit

- 1 teaspoon vanilla flavor

Instructions:

1. In a large bowl, add all ingredients and mix well.

2. Roll the dough into small balls (about 1 inch in diameter).

3. Place the balls on a baking sheet lined with parchment paper and chill for at least 30 minutes.

4. Store in an airtight jar in the refrigerator for up to a week.

2. Hummus and Veggie Sticks

Hummus paired with fresh veggies makes a crunchy and satisfying snack packed with fiber, protein, and healthy fats.

Ingredients:

- 1 cup hummus (store-bought or homemade)
- 1 carrot, cut into sticks
- 1 cucumber, cut into sticks
- 1 bell pepper, cut into strips
- A handful of cherry tomatoes

Instructions:

1. Arrange the veggie sticks and cherry tomatoes on a plate.
2. Serve with a bowl of hummus for dipping.
3. Enjoy as a refreshing and healthy snack.

3. Avocado Toast

Avocado toast is a trendy snack that's both delicious and healthy. It's quick to prepare and can be topped with different ingredients to suit your taste.

Ingredients:

- 1 slice whole grain or sourdough bread

- 1/2 ripe avocado

- A squeeze of lemon juice

- Salt and pepper to taste

- Optional toppings: cherry tomatoes, radish pieces, microgreens, or a poached egg

Instructions:

1. Toast the bread to your desired amount of crispiness.

2. While the bread is heating, mash the avocado in a small bowl and season with lemon juice, salt, and pepper.

3. Spread the mashed avocado on the toast.

4. Add your favorite toppings and enjoy instantly.

4. Fruit and Nut Mix

A homemade fruit and nut mix is a handy and nutritious snack that provides a balance of healthy fats, protein, and carbohydrates.

Ingredients:

- 1/2 cup raw almonds

- 1/2 cup raw cashews

- 1/4 cup pumpkin seeds

- 1/4 cup dried cherries or raisins

- 1/4 cup dark chocolate chips (optional)

Instructions:

1. In a large bowl, add all ingredients and mix well.

2. Store the mix in an airtight jar or portion into small bags for on-the-go snacking.

5. Smoothie

A smoothie is a flexible and delicious way to pack a lot of nutrients into a single snack. Choose a range of fruits, vegetables, and protein sources to create a balanced blend.

Ingredients:
- 1 cup spinach or kale
- 1 orange
- 1/2 cup frozen berries
- 1/2 cup Greek yogurt or a scoop of protein powder

- 1 tablespoon chia seeds

- 1 cup unsweetened almond milk or water

Instructions:

1. Add all ingredients to a blender.

2. Blend until smooth and creamy.

3. Pour into a glass and enjoy instantly.

6. Cottage Cheese and Pineapple

Cottage cheese paired with pineapple is a high-protein snack that's sweet and filling. The combination of protein and fruit makes it a great choice for any time of the day.

Ingredients:

- 1 cup low-fat cottage cheese

- 1/2 cup fresh or canned pineapple chunks (in juice, not sauce)

- A sprinkle of cinnamon (optional)

Instructions:

1. In a bowl, mix the cottage cheese and pineapple chunks.

2. Sprinkle with cinnamon if wanted.

3. Enjoy quickly.

Healthy snacking doesn't have to be difficult or time-consuming. By making smart choices and having a range of nutritious options available, you can enjoy satisfying snacks that support your health and well-being. With the recipe ideas given, you'll have plenty of delicious and nutritious snacks to keep you fueled and satisfied throughout the day.

Day 6: Stress Management and Emotional Eating

Welcome to Day 6 of your two-week guide to breaking free from the cycle of cravings, boosting your metabolism, and reclaiming your energy. Today, we look into stress management and emotional eating—two interlinked factors that greatly impact your eating habits and overall health. By learning effective techniques to lower stress and understanding the dynamics of emotional eating, you can gain better control over your dietary choices and improve your well-being.

Techniques to Reduce Stress

Stress is an inevitable part of life, but how you handle it can make a big difference in your health and eating behaviors. Here are some practical methods to help you reduce stress:

1. Mindfulness and Meditation

Mindfulness includes staying present and fully engaging with the current moment without judgment. Meditation is a practice that helps cultivate mindfulness, and it has been shown to reduce stress and anxiety greatly.

How to Practice:

- Mindful Breathing: Sit or lie down in a relaxed position. Close your eyes and take slow, deep breaths, focused on the sensation of the air entering and leaving your body. When your mind wanders, gently bring your attention back to your breath.

- Body Scan Meditation: Lie down and focus on each part of your body, starting from your toes and going up to your head. Notice any sensations, tension, or pain, and breathe into those areas.

- Guided Meditation: Use apps or online tools that offer guided meditation sessions, which can help you relax and reduce stress.

2. Physical Activity

Exercise is a great stress reliever. It helps release endorphins, which are natural mood lifters, and lowers the levels of stress hormones like cortisol.

How to Incorporate:

- Regular Exercise: Aim for at least 30 minutes of moderate activity most days of the week. Activities like walking, running, swimming, or cycling can be very efficient.

- Yoga: This combines physical movement with mindfulness and breathing exercises, making it an excellent choice for stress relief.

- Short Breaks: Even short bursts of physical exercise, like a 10-minute walk, can help clear your mind and reduce stress.

3. Adequate Sleep

Getting enough quality sleep is important for managing stress. Lack of sleep can exacerbate stress and make it harder to deal with daily challenges.

Tips for Better Sleep:

- Consistent Schedule: Go to bed and wake up at the same time every day, even on weekends.

- Sleep Environment: Make sure your bedroom is suitable to sleep—cool, dark, and quiet.

- Limit Screen Time: Avoid screens (phones, tablets, computers) for at least an hour before bedtime, as the blue light can interfere with your sleep routine.

4. Healthy Eating

Nourishing your body with balanced, healthy meals can improve your happiness and energy levels, helping you cope with stress more effectively.

Strategies:

- Balanced Diet: Focus on whole foods like fruits, veggies, whole grains, lean proteins, and healthy fats.

- Avoid Stimulants: Limit your intake of coffee and sugar, which can cause spikes and crashes in your energy and mood.

- Hydration: Drink plenty of water throughout the day to stay refreshed.

5. **Social Support**

Connecting with others can provide emotional support and help you handle stress. Sharing your thoughts and feelings with friends or family members can be very helpful.

Ways to Connect:

- Regular Catch-Ups: Make time for regular phone calls, video chats, or meet-ups with loved ones.
- Join Groups: Participate in community groups or clubs that interest you.
- Seek Professional Help: If stress becomes overwhelming, try speaking with a therapist or counselor.

6. Relaxation Techniques

Incorporate relaxation methods into your daily routine to help your body and mind unwind.

Methods:

- Deep Breathing: Practice deep breathing exercises to help calm your nervous system.

- Progressive Muscle Relaxation: Tense and then slowly release each muscle group in your body, starting from your toes and going up to your head.

- Visualization: Imagine a peaceful scene or place that makes you feel relaxed and happy.

Understanding Emotional Eating

Emotional eating is the practice of using food to cope with feelings rather than to satisfy hunger. Stress, sadness, boredom, and even happiness can cause emotional eating. Understanding the underlying causes and developing healthier coping strategies can help you break free from this cycle.

What is Emotional Eating?

Emotional eating involves consuming food in response to emotional wants rather than physical hunger. It often leads to eating high-calorie, sugary, or fatty foods that provide brief comfort but can result in feelings of guilt and shame later.

Common Triggers:

- Stress: High levels of stress can boost the hormone cortisol, which may trigger cravings for sugary and fatty foods.

- Boredom: Eating can be a way to fill time or provide a sense of purpose.

- Emotional States: Sadness, loneliness, anger, and even happiness can lead to emotional eating.

- Social Influences: Social situations and peer pressure can also cause emotional eating.

How to Recognize Emotional Eating:

Identifying whether you're eating out of hunger or feeling is the first step in addressing emotional eating. Here are some signs:

- Sudden Cravings: Emotional hunger often comes on suddenly and is special to certain comfort foods.

- Mindless Eating: Eating without really paying attention to the food or without feeling pleasure.

- Eating When Full: Consuming food even when you're not physically hungry.

- Feelings of Guilt: Feeling sorry or ashamed after eating.

Strategies to Overcome Emotional Eating

1. Identify Triggers

Keep a food log to track what you eat, when you eat, and how you feel before and after eating. This can help you spot patterns and triggers of emotional eating.

2. Find Alternatives

Develop healthy coping strategies to deal with emotions instead of turning to food.

Alternatives:

- Physical action: Go for a walk, run, or engage in any physical action you enjoy.
- Creative Outlets: Engage in hobbies like painting, writing, or playing an instrument.
- Relaxation Techniques: Practice meditation, deep breathing, or take a warm bath.

3. Practice Mindful Eating

Mindful eating can help you stay present and aware during meals, reducing the chance of emotional eating.

Techniques:

- Eat Slowly: Take your time to savor each bite and chew fully.

- Focus on Your Food: Remove distractions like TV or phones while eating.

- Listen to Your Body: Pay attention to your hunger and fullness feelings.

4. Build a Support System

Having a support system can help you manage emotions more effectively and lessen the reliance on food for comfort.

Support Strategies:

- Talk it Out: Share your thoughts with a trusted friend or family member.

- Join a Support Group: Consider joining a group for emotional eaters or stress management.

- Professional Help: Seek advice from a therapist or counselor to address underlying emotional issues.

5. Plan and Prepare

Planning and making your meals and snacks can help you make healthier choices and avoid impulsive eating.

Tips:

- Meal Prep: Prepare healthy meals and snacks in advance to have nutritious options easily available.

-Healthy Alternatives: Keep healthy snacks like fruits, veggies, nuts, and yogurt on hand.

- Stay Hydrated: Drink plenty of water throughout the day, as thirst can sometimes be confused for hunger.

Day 7: Weekly Reflection and Adjustment

Congratulations on reaching Day 7 of your journey to break free from the cycle of cravings, boost your metabolism, and reclaim your energy. Today marks an important milestone: a day devoted to reflection and adjustment. Reflecting on your progress and making necessary adjustments are crucial steps in ensuring your ongoing success and longevity of the changes you're making. This process allows you to celebrate your achievements, identify areas for improvement, and refine your strategies going forward.

Reviewing Your Progress

Reviewing your progress is a powerful practice that can provide valuable insights into your journey. It's a time to acknowledge what you've accomplished, recognize the challenges you've met, and understand how your body and mind have responded to the changes. Here's a structured method to reviewing your progress:

1. Reflect on Your Goals

Begin by revisiting the goals you set at the start of this trip. What were your goals for these two weeks? Whether your goals were related to reducing cravings, improving your eating habits, increasing your energy levels, or something else, it's important to measure your progress against these benchmarks.

Questions to Ask:

- Have I been able to lessen my cravings? If so, how?

- Have my eating habits improved? In what ways?

- Do I feel more energized and vitalized?

- Am I feeling any positive changes in my mood or overall well-being?

2. Celebrate Your Achievements

Recognizing and celebrating your successes, no matter how small, is important for motivation and self-encouragement. Reflect on the positive changes you've made and the times when you stayed committed to your goals.

Areas to Celebrate:

- Times when you successfully managed urges.

- Healthy food choices you've made.

- Instances where you practiced careful eating.

- Any physical activities or exercises you added into your routine.

3. Identify Challenges and Obstacles

Understanding the challenges you've faced can help you develop strategies to overcome them in the future. Reflect on any difficulties or setbacks you experienced during the week.

Questions to Consider:

- Were there moments when cravings were particularly strong? What triggered them?

- Did you find it challenging to stick to healthy eating? Why?

- Were there times when stress or emotions affect your eating habits?

- How did you handle social events involving food?

4. Assess Physical and Emotional Changes

Pay attention to any physical or mental changes you've noticed. These changes can provide signs about how your body and mind are responding to your new habits.

Areas to Reflect On:

- Changes in energy levels throughout the day.

- Improvements in stomach or physical comfort.

- Shifts in mood or stress levels.

- Any weight changes or differences in how your clothes fit.

Making Necessary Adjustments

After reflecting on your progress, it's time to make adjustments to improve your journey further. Making adjustments ensures that you're continually refining your method based on what's working and what isn't. Here's how to successfully make necessary adjustments:

1. Set New Goals or Refine Existing Ones

Based on your reflections, you may find that your original goals need adjustment. Setting new goals or refining old ones can provide renewed focus and direction.

Considerations:

- If you achieved your original goals, consider setting new, more challenging goals.

- If you didn't fully achieve your goals, refine them to be more detailed, realistic, or attainable.

- Incorporate any new insights or goals that emerged during your reflection.

2. Develop Strategies for Overcoming Challenges

Identifying challenges is only the first step; developing strategies to beat them is crucial. Consider practical solutions and proactive steps to address the obstacles you've faced.

Strategies:

- Cravings Management: If cravings were a major challenge, explore additional strategies such as drinking water before eating, distracting yourself with a non-food activity, or trying alternative snacks.

- Healthy Eating: If sticking to healthy eating was tough, plan and prepare meals in advance, keep healthy snacks on hand, and create a shopping list to avoid impulse purchases.

- Stress and Emotional Eating: If stress or emotions influenced your eating, incorporate stress-management techniques like mindfulness, meditation, or physical exercise into your daily routine.

3. Enhance Your Support System

Having a strong support system can greatly impact your success. Consider ways to enhance or grow your support network.

Actions to Take:
- Share your goals and progress with friends or family members who can provide support and accountability.

- Join a support group or community, either in person or online, where you can meet with others who share similar goals.

- Consider seeking guidance from a professional, such as a nutritionist or therapist, if you need extra support.

4. Adjust Your Routine

Your daily routine plays a significant role in your ability to keep healthy habits. Adjusting your routine can help make it easier to stay on track.

Routine Adjustments:
- Meal Timing: Adjust your meal timing to better match with your hunger cues and daily schedule.

- Exercise: Incorporate regular physical exercise that you enjoy and can realistically maintain.

- Sleep: Ensure you're getting adequate sleep by establishing a consistent bedtime routine and making a conducive sleep environment.

5. Monitor and Reflect Regularly

Reflection and change should be ongoing processes. Regularly monitoring your progress and reflecting on your experiences can help you stay focused and make timely changes.

Monitoring Tips:

- Keep a Journal: Maintain a journal to track your food intake, physical exercise, moods, and reflections. This can provide useful insights over time.

- Set Regular Check-Ins: Schedule regular check-ins with yourself to review your progress and change your goals and strategies as needed.

- Celebrate Milestones: Acknowledge and celebrate milestones along the way to stay motivated and happy.

6. Stay Flexible and Compassionate

Finally, remember that flexibility and self-compassion are important components of any successful journey. Life is unpredictable, and setbacks are a normal part of the process. Treat yourself with kindness and understanding, and be ready to adapt as needed.

Mindset Tips:

- Self-Compassion: Treat yourself with the same kindness and understanding that you would offer a friend. Acknowledge that everyone faces challenges and that setbacks are chances for growth.

- Adaptability: Be open to trying new methods and making changes as you learn more about what works best for you.

- Positive Thinking: Focus on your growth and the positive changes you're making, rather than dwelling on any perceived failures.

Day 7 is a pivotal point in your two-week journey, giving a chance to pause, reflect, and adjust your course. By reviewing your progress and making necessary changes, you're setting yourself up for continued success and sustainability. Celebrate your successes, learn from your challenges, and refine your strategies to better align with your goals and needs. Remember, this journey is about making lasting, positive changes that support your overall health and well-being. Keep moving forward with confidence and determination, and embrace each day as a chance to grow and thrive.

Week 2: Boosting Your Metabolism

Day 8: The Role of Exercise

Congratulations on making it to Week 2 of your journey towards breaking free from cravings, boosting your metabolism, and reclaiming your energy. This week, our attention shifts to enhancing your metabolism. Today, we will explore the significant role exercise plays in this process and discuss different types of exercise that are particularly beneficial for metabolic health.

How Exercise Affects Metabolism

To understand how exercise impacts metabolism, it's important to grasp the basics of what metabolism is. Metabolism refers to all the chemical processes that occur within your body to keep life. This includes converting food into energy, growing and repairing tissues, and eliminating waste products. Exercise affects these processes in several profound ways:

1. Increases Caloric Expenditure

When you exercise, your body needs more energy to sustain physical activity. This higher energy demand raises your metabolic rate, meaning you burn more calories both during and after the workout. The length and intensity of your exercise determine how much your metabolic rate increases. High-intensity workouts tend to cause a more significant and longer-lasting boost in metabolism, known as the afterburn effect or excess post-exercise oxygen consumption (EPOC).

2. Enhances Muscle Mass

Muscle tissue is metabolically active, meaning it needs more energy to maintain compared to fat tissue. By engaging in strength training and other types of resistance exercise, you can increase your muscle mass. More muscle mass translates to a higher resting metabolic rate (RMR), which is the number of calories your body burns at rest. This means you will burn more calories throughout the day, even when you are not moving.

3. Improves Hormonal Balance

Regular exercise positively changes hormone levels that regulate metabolism. For instance:

- Insulin Sensitivity: Exercise improves your cells' sensitivity to insulin, allowing them to use glucose more effectively and reducing the chance of storing excess glucose as fat.

- Growth Hormone: Physical movement stimulates the release of growth hormone, which plays a role in muscle growth, fat metabolism, and overall metabolic health.

- Adiponectin: Exercise increases the production of adiponectin, a hormone that improves your muscles' ability to use carbohydrates for energy, boosts metabolism, and aids in fat burning.

4. Enhances Mitochondrial Function

Mitochondria are the powerhouses of your cells, responsible for making energy. Regular exercise improves both the number and efficiency of mitochondria in your muscle cells, leading to better energy production and higher metabolic efficiency.

5. Reduces Visceral Fat

Exercise helps lower visceral fat, which is the harmful fat stored around your internal organs. Excess visceral fat is linked to different metabolic disorders, including insulin resistance and inflammation. By reducing this type of fat, exercise helps improve your metabolic health.

Types of Beneficial Exercise

To maximize the metabolic benefits of exercise, it's important to add a variety of physical activities into your routine. Here are some types of exercise that are particularly helpful for boosting metabolism:

1. Cardiovascular Exercise

Cardiovascular or aerobic exercise includes tasks that increase your heart rate and breathing. This type of exercise is great for burning calories and improving cardiovascular health.

Examples:

- Running or Jogging: These activities can be done outdoors or on a machine and are effective for burning calories and improving heart health.

- Cycling: Whether on a stationary bike or riding outdoors, cycling is a low-impact workout that boosts your metabolism.

- Swimming: Swimming uses multiple muscle groups and provides a full-body workout, making it an excellent choice for boosting metabolism.

- Brisk Walking: Walking at a brisk pace is accessible to most people and can significantly add to daily calorie expenditure.

2. High-Intensity Interval Training (HIIT)

HIIT involves short bursts of intense exercise followed by times of rest or low-intensity exercise. This type of workout is highly beneficial for increasing metabolic rate and promoting fat loss.

Benefits:
- Afterburn Effect: HIIT workouts create a significant afterburn effect, leading to increased calorie burn even after the workout is finished.

- Time-Efficient: HIIT sessions are usually shorter in duration but offer comparable benefits to longer, moderate-intensity workouts.

Examples:

- Sprint Intervals: Alternating between running and walking or jogging.

- Circuit Training: Performing a number of strength exercises with minimal rest in between.

- Tabata: A specific type of HIIT that includes 20 seconds of intense exercise followed by 10 seconds of rest, repeated for 4 minutes.

3. Strength Training

Strength or resistance training focuses on building and keeping muscle mass. This type of exercise is important for increasing resting metabolic rate and overall metabolic health.

Benefits:

- Muscle Growth: Promotes muscle growth, which increases metabolic rate.
- Bone Health: Strengthens bones and lowers the risk of osteoporosis.

Examples:

- Weightlifting: Using free weights or weight machines to perform movements like squats, deadlifts, and bench presses.

- Bodyweight Exercises: Utilizing your own body weight for support, such as push-ups, pull-ups, and lunges.

- Resistance Bands: Incorporating resistance bands into your workout to add variety and challenge.

4. Flexibility and Balance Exercises

While not directly linked to metabolic rate, flexibility and balance exercises are important for overall fitness and injury prevention. These movements complement your metabolic-boosting workouts by improving range of motion, posture, and coordination.

Examples:

- Yoga: Combines flexibility, strength, and mindfulness. Certain types of yoga, like power yoga, can also provide a cardio workout.

- Pilates: Focuses on core strength, flexibility, and total body conditioning.

- Stretching: Regular stretching routines help keep muscle flexibility and prevent injuries.

5. Non-Exercise Activity Thermogenesis (NEAT)

NEAT includes all the physical activities that are not organized exercise, such as walking to work, gardening, cleaning, and even fidgeting. These activities add significantly to your daily calorie expenditure and overall metabolic rate.

Strategies to Increase NEAT:

- Take the Stairs: Opt for stairs instead of lifts or escalators whenever possible.

- Walk More: Incorporate walking into your daily routine, such as walking during phone calls or parking further away from exits.

- Active Breaks: Take short, frequent breaks to move around if you have a sedentary job.

- Household Chores: Engage in activities like cleaning, gardening, or organizing to stay busy throughout the day.

Exercise plays a pivotal role in boosting your metabolism, enhancing your body's ability to burn calories, build muscle, and keep overall health. By understanding how exercise affects metabolism and adding a variety of physical activities into your routine, you can optimize your metabolic rate and achieve your health goals. Remember, the key is consistency and variety—mixing cardiovascular exercise, HIIT, strength training, flexibility exercises, and increasing NEAT will ensure you get the most complete metabolic benefits. Keep pushing forward with determination, and you'll continue to see improvements in your energy levels, body composition, and general vitality.

Day 9: High-Intensity Interval Training (HIIT)

Welcome to Day 9 of your two-week guide to boosting your metabolism and reclaiming your energy. Today, we're going into the world of High-Intensity Interval Training (HIIT). HIIT is famous for its efficiency and effectiveness in improving cardiovascular health, burning fat, and boosting metabolism. Let's explore what HIIT is, how it works, and some sample workouts you can add into your routine.

What is HIIT?

High-Intensity Interval Training (HIIT) is a form of exercise that alternates between short bursts of intense activity and times of lower-intensity recovery or rest. The key feature of HIIT is the intensity during the work intervals, which should be high enough to push your boundaries. The recovery times allow your body to partially recover before the next burst of intense activity, making it possible to maintain a high level of effort throughout the workout.

The Science Behind HIIT

HIIT leverages the principle of EPOC (Excess Post-Exercise Oxygen Consumption), widely referred to as the afterburn effect. This means that after finishing an HIIT workout, your body continues to burn calories at an elevated rate as it works to return to its normal resting state. This effect can last for hours, greatly increasing the total calorie expenditure from the workout.

Benefits of HIIT

1. Efficiency: HIIT workouts are generally short, often ranging from 15 to 30 minutes, making them ideal for those with busy schedules.

2. Calorie Burn: The high intensity of HIIT leads to a large calorie burn during and after the workout.

3. Cardiovascular Health: HIIT improves cardiovascular fitness by pushing your heart and lungs during intense intervals.

4. Fat Loss:By boosting your metabolism and promoting the afterburn effect, HIIT is useful for reducing body fat.

5. Muscle Retention: Unlike steady-state cardio, HIIT helps maintain muscle mass while burning fat.

6. Variety: HIIT can be applied to different forms of exercise, from running and cycling to bodyweight exercises and weight training.

Sample Workouts

To get you started with HIIT, here are some sample workouts that cater to different fitness levels and tastes. Each workout includes a warm-up, work sprints, and a cool-down. Always start with a 5-10 minute warm-up to prepare your body and end with a 5-10 minute cool-down to help recovery.

1. Beginner HIIT Workout

This workout is meant for those new to HIIT or returning to exercise after a break. The work intervals are challenging but manageable, with suitable recovery breaks.

Warm-Up:
- 5 minutes of light running or brisk walking
- Dynamic stretches (leg swings, arm circles, hip circles)

Workout:
- 30 seconds of jumping jacks
- 30 seconds of rest
- 30 seconds of bodyweight squats
- 30 seconds of rest
- 30 seconds of mountain climbers
- 30 seconds of rest

- 30 seconds of push-ups (adjust to knees if needed)

- 30 seconds of rest

Repeat the circle 3-4 times.

Cool-Down:

- 5 minutes of walking

- Static stretches (hamstrings, quads, shoulders)

2. Intermediate HIIT Workout

This workout ramps up the intensity and includes exercises that test multiple muscle groups. It's great for those who have some experience with HIIT.

Warm-Up:

- 5 minutes of jogging

- Dynamic stretches (high knees, butt kicks, torso bends)

Workout:

- 40 seconds of burpees

- 20 seconds of rest

- 40 seconds of alternate lunges

- 20 seconds of rest

- 40 seconds of high knees

- 20 seconds of rest

- 40 seconds of plank to push-up

- 20 seconds of rest

Repeat the circle 4-5 times.

Cool-Down:

- 5 minutes of slow running or walking

- Static stretches (calves, hip flexors, chest)

3. Advanced HIIT Workout

This high-intensity workout is meant for those who are well-acquainted with HIIT and seek a serious challenge. The intervals are longer, and the exercises demand more work.

Warm-Up:

- 5 minutes of running

- Dynamic stretches (lunges with a twist, arm swings, hip openers)

Workout:

- 50 seconds of sprinting or fast running

- 10 seconds of rest

- 50 seconds of jump squats

- 10 seconds of rest

- 50 seconds of bicycle crunches

- 10 seconds of rest

-50 seconds of kettlebell swings (if possible)

- 10 seconds of rest

Repeat the circle 5-6 times.

Cool-Down:

- 5-10 minutes of light running or walking

- Static stretches (glutes, biceps, lower back)

4. Low-Impact HIIT Workout

For those who need a low-impact option, this workout offers the benefits of HIIT without the high-impact movements that can stress joints.

Warm-Up:

- 5 minutes of walking in place or light cycling

- Dynamic stretches (leg lifts, shoulder rolls, side bends)

Workout:

- 30 seconds of walking in place with high knees

- 30 seconds of rest

- 30 seconds of step-ups (using a strong chair or bench)

- 30 seconds of rest

- 30 seconds of low-impact side-to-side lunges

- 30 seconds of rest

- 30 seconds of standing punches

- 30 seconds of rest

Repeat the circle 3-4 times.

Cool-Down:

- 5 minutes of easy walking

- Static stretches (hamstrings, calves, arms)

5. HIIT with Equipment

Incorporating equipment can add variety and energy to your HIIT workouts. This sample uses a jump rope, dumbbells, and a medicine ball.

Warm-Up:

- 5 minutes of jump rope or brisk walking

- Dynamic stretches (jumping jacks, arm circles, hip circles)

Workout:

- 40 seconds of jump rope

- 20 seconds of rest

- 40 seconds of dumbbell lifts (squat to press)

- 20 seconds of rest

- 40 seconds of medicine ball hits

- 20 seconds of rest

- 40 seconds of rogue rows (with dumbbells)

- 20 seconds of rest

Repeat the circle 4-5 times.

Cool-Down:

- 5 minutes of light running or walking

- Static stretches (quads, hips, shoulders)

High-Intensity Interval Training (HIIT) is a strong tool for boosting metabolism, burning fat, and improving cardiovascular fitness. Its versatility allows you to tailor workouts to your fitness level and preferences, ensuring you can constantly challenge yourself and make progress. Whether you're a beginner easing into exercise or an advanced athlete trying to push your limits, there's an HIIT workout for you.

Remember to listen to your body and change the intensity and duration of your workouts as needed. Consistency is key, and adding HIIT into your routine, even a few times a week, can lead to significant changes in your overall health and fitness.

Day 10: Strength Training Essentials

Welcome to Day 10 of your two-week journey to break free from cravings, boost your metabolism, and reclaim your energy. Today's focus is on strength training, a crucial component of a well-rounded fitness routine. Strength training not only builds muscle but also improves overall health in myriad ways.

Benefits of Strength Training

1. Increased Muscle Mass and Strength

The main benefit of strength training is, of course, the development of muscle mass and strength. As you engage in resistance exercises, your muscles adapt by getting stronger and larger. This increased muscle mass adds to a more toned and defined appearance, enhancing physical aesthetics and performance.

2. Enhanced Metabolic Rate

Muscle tissue is metabolically active, meaning it needs more energy (calories) to maintain than fat tissue. By increasing your muscle mass through strength training, you increase your resting metabolic rate (RMR), which is the number of calories your body burns at rest. This enhanced metabolic rate helps with weight control and fat loss, even when you're not actively exercising.

3. Improved Bone Density

Strength training puts stress on your bones, stimulating bone-forming cells and enhancing bone density. This is particularly important for preventing osteoporosis and lowering the risk of fractures, especially as you age.

4. Better Joint Health and Stability

Strengthening the muscles around your joints provides better support and stability, reducing the risk of injuries and improving general joint health. This is beneficial for keeping mobility and independence, especially in later years.

5. Enhanced Functional Fitness

Functional fitness refers to the ability to perform everyday tasks with ease. Strength training improves your ability to carry out daily tasks, such as lifting groceries, climbing stairs, and playing with children, by enhancing general strength and endurance.

6. Improved Mental Health

Engaging in strength training has been shown to have good effects on mental health. It can lower symptoms of anxiety and depression, boost mood, and improve cognitive function. The sense of accomplishment and increased self-esteem that comes from achieving strength-related goals further add to mental well-being.

7. Better Blood Sugar Control

Strength training improves insulin sensitivity, allowing your muscles to use glucose more effectively. This helps in regulating blood sugar levels and can be particularly beneficial for individuals with type 2 diabetes or those at risk of getting it.

8. Cardiovascular Health

While strength training is generally known for building muscle, it also has positive effects on cardiovascular health. Regular strength training can reduce blood pressure, improve cholesterol levels, and boost overall heart health.

Beginner Routines

If you're new to strength training, it's important to start with a structured routine that focuses on building a solid foundation. Here are a few beginner routines that target major muscle groups and help you build proper form and technique.

Routine 1: Full-Body Beginner Workout

This full-body workout is meant to be performed 2-3 times a week, with at least one rest day in between sessions. It targets all the major muscle groups and can be done using minimal tools, such as dumbbells or resistance bands.

Warm-Up:

- 5-10 minutes of light exercise (e.g., brisk walking, jogging, jumping jacks)

- Dynamic stretches (e.g., leg swings, arm circles, hip circles)

Workout:

1. Squats (Bodyweight or with tools)

- Sets: 3

- Reps: 12-15

- Tips: Keep your feet shoulder-width apart, chest up, and bottom down as if sitting in a chair. Push through your heels to stand back up.

2. Push-Ups (Modify to knees if needed)

- Sets: 3

- Reps: 10-12

- Tips: Keep your body in a straight line from head to heels, lower down until your chest almost hits the floor, and push back up.

3. Bent-Over Rows (With dumbbells or training bands)
- Sets: 3
- Reps: 12-15
- Tips: Hinge at your hips with a slight bend in your knees, keep your back flat, and pull the weights towards your hips.

4. Plank
- Sets: 3
- Duration: 20-30 seconds
- Tips: Maintain a straight line from head to feet, keep your core tight, and avoid sagging your hips.

5. Lunges (Bodyweight or with arms)

- Sets: 3

- Reps: 10-12 per leg

- Tips: Step forward with one leg, lower your hips until both knees are at 90-degree angles, and push back up through your front heel.

6. Dumbbell Shoulder Press

- Sets: 3

- Reps: 12-15

- Tips: Hold the dumbbells at shoulder height, press them overhead while keeping your core engaged, and bring them back down.

Cool-Down:

- 5-10 minutes of light stretching (e.g., hamstrings, quadriceps, shoulders, forearms)

Routine 2: Upper/Lower Split

This plan splits the workouts into upper body and lower body days, allowing for focused training and more recovery time for each muscle group. Perform each workout twice a week, with at least one rest day between rounds.

Upper Body Workout:

Warm-Up:
- 5-10 minutes of light exercise (e.g., brisk walking, jogging, arm circles)

Workout:
1. Push-Ups (Modify to knees if needed)
- Sets: 3

- Reps: 10-12

2. Bent-Over Rows (With dumbbells or exercise bands)

- Sets: 3

- Reps: 12-15

3. Dumbbell Shoulder Press

- Sets: 3

- Reps: 12-15

4. Bicep Curls (With dumbbells)

- Sets: 3

- Reps: 12-15

5. Tricep Dips (Using a chair or bench)

- Sets: 3

- Reps: 10-12

6. Plank - Sets: 3 - Duration: 20-30 seconds

Cool-Down:

- 5-10 minutes of light stretching (e.g., chest, shoulders, arms)

Lower Body Workout:

Warm-Up:

- 5-10 minutes of light exercise (e.g., brisk walking, jogging, leg swings)

Workout:

1. Squats (Bodyweight or with tools)
- Sets: 3
- Reps: 12-15

2. Lunges (Bodyweight or with arms)

- Sets: 3

- Reps: 10-12 per leg

3. Glute Bridges

- Sets: 3 - Reps: 15-20

- Tips: Lie on your back with knees bent, lift your hips towards the sky, squeeze your glutes at the top, and lower back down.

4. Leg Press (Using a machine if possible)

- Sets: 3

- Reps: 12-15

5. Calf Raises (Bodyweight or with dumbbells)

- Sets: 3

- Reps: 15-20

- Tips: Stand with feet shoulder-width apart, raise your heels off the ground, and lower back down slowly.

6. Side Leg Raises (With or without ankle weights)
- Sets: 3
- Reps: 15-20 per leg
- Tips: Lie on your side, lift your top leg towards the sky, and lower it back down.

Cool-Down:
- 5-10 minutes of light stretching (e.g., hamstrings, quads, calves)

Tips for Success

1. Focus on Form

Proper form is crucial to avoid injuries and ensure you are effectively targeting the intended muscles. Take the time to learn the right techniques for each exercise. If possible, work with a trainer or watch instructional movies to understand proper alignment and movement.

2. Start Light

Begin with lighter weights or just your body weight to get comfortable with the movements. As you become more confident and your strength improves, gradually raise the resistance to continue challenging your muscles.

3. Rest and Recover

Give your muscles time to recover between strength training workouts. Aim for at least one rest day between workouts that target the same muscle groups. During rest days, focus on light activities such as walking or stretching to aid healing.

4. Stay Consistent

Consistency is key to seeing growth. Aim to add strength training into your routine 2-3 times a week. Over time, you'll notice improvements in your strength, muscle tone, and general fitness.

5. Listen to Your Body

Pay attention to how your body feels during and after workouts. If you experience pain (as opposed to normal muscle soreness), stop the exercise and seek a healthcare professional if necessary. It's important to push yourself, but not at the price of your health.

Strength training is a strong tool for enhancing your physical and mental health. By building muscle, increasing metabolic rate, and improving physical fitness, you set the stage for long-term well-being. Start with the beginner routines provided, focus on proper form, and gradually increase your intensity as you improve.

Day 11: Cardio for a Healthy Heart

Welcome to Day 11 of your journey to improve your health and vitality. Today, we're focused on cardiovascular exercise, commonly referred to as cardio. Cardio is important for maintaining a healthy heart, improving overall fitness, and supporting weight management. In this session, we'll explore various cardio choices and provide practical tips for incorporating cardio into your routine.

Cardio Options

Cardiovascular exercise includes any activity that raises your heart rate and improves blood circulation throughout the body. Here are some popular and effective cardio choices to consider:

1. Running and Jogging

Running and jogging are simple, accessible forms of cardio that can be done almost anywhere. They are excellent for improving cardiovascular health, burning calories, and strengthening endurance.

Pros:

- No special equipment needed beyond good running shoes
- Can be done outdoors or on a bike
- Scalable intensity, from light running to sprinting

Cons:

- High impact, which may not be ideal for everyone, especially those with joint issues

- Requires access to safe, suitable running tracks or a treadmill

2. Walking

Walking is a low-impact, highly accessible form of cardio that's good for people of all fitness levels. It's particularly helpful for beginners or those recovering from injuries.

Pros:
- Gentle on the joints
- Can be done anywhere, indoors or outdoors
- Easy to add into daily routines (e.g., walking to work or during breaks)

Cons:

- Less intense than other forms of cardio, so it may need to be done for longer durations to gain equal benefits

3. Cycling

Cycling, whether on a stationary bike or outdoors, is an effective cardiovascular workout that's also gentle on the knees. It's great for building lower body strength while improving heart health.

Pros:
- Low-impact, ideal for people with joint issues
- Can be done indoors or outdoors
- Great for building leg strength and endurance
Cons:

- Requires a bike or access to a stationary bike
- Outdoor riding may depend on weather conditions

4. Swimming

Swimming is a full-body workout that's highly useful for cardiovascular fitness. It's an excellent choice for those with joint issues, as it's a low-impact activity.

Pros:
- Low-impact and gentle on the joints
- Full-body workout, engaging various muscle groups
- Can be relaxing and stress-relieving

Cons:

-Requires access to a pool

- May not be suitable for those who are not strong swimmers

5. Rowing

Rowing, whether on a machine or in the water, provides a full-body workout that stresses both cardiovascular fitness and muscular strength.

Pros:
- Low-impact, lowering strain on joints
- Full-body workout, engaging upper body, core, and legs
- Can be done indoors on a rowing machine

Cons:

- Requires a rowing machine or access to a boat and river

- Proper technique is important to avoid injury

6. Dancing

Dancing is a fun and lively way to get your cardio workout. Various types of dance, from Zumba to ballroom, offer cardiovascular benefits while allowing you to enjoy music and movement.

Pros:

- Fun and engaging, making it easier to stick with

- Can be done in a group setting, improving social interaction

- Great for coordination and balance

Cons:

- May require access to classes or sufficient space at home

- Intensity can change, so it's important to choose styles that elevate heart rate

7. Jump Rope

Jumping rope is a great high-intensity cardio workout that can be done almost anywhere. It's great for improving coordination, agility, and cardiovascular stamina.

Pros:

- Highly portable and inexpensive equipment

- Burns a large number of calories in a short time - Improves coordination and agility

Cons:

- High-impact, which may not be ideal for everyone

- Requires some skill and practice to perform effectively

Cardiovascular exercise is a cornerstone of a healthy living. It strengthens your heart, improves your general fitness, and supports mental well-being. By exploring different cardio choices and incorporating them into your routine, you can enjoy the many benefits of a healthy heart and an active life.

Day 12: The Importance of Rest and Recovery

Welcome to Day 12 of your two-week journey to boost your metabolism, break free from cravings, and reclaim your energy. Today's focus is on an often-overlooked but critical part of health and fitness: rest and recovery. Proper recovery allows your body to heal, adapt, and grow stronger, while adequate sleep is important for overall well-being.

Why Recovery Matters

Recovery is the process through which your body repairs and adapts to the stress caused by exercise and daily activities. It includes physical, mental, and emotional components, all of which are essential for achieving optimal health and performance. Here are key reasons why healing is vital:

1. Muscle Repair and Growth

During exercise, especially strength training, you make small tears in your muscle fibers. Recovery allows these fibers to repair and grow stronger, leading to increased muscle mass and better physical performance.

2. Injury Prevention

Adequate recovery lowers the risk of overuse injuries, which occur when the body does not have enough time to heal between workouts. Rest days and correct recovery techniques help prevent strains, sprains, and other injuries.

3. Improved Performance

Without proper recovery, your performance can plateau or even decline. Recovery helps your body to replenish energy stores, repair tissues, and restore balance, leading to better performance in future workouts.

4. Hormonal Balance

Exercise impacts different hormones, including cortisol (the stress hormone) and growth hormone. Proper recovery helps regulate these hormones, ensuring they stay balanced and contribute to overall health rather than detracting from it.

5. Mental Health

Recovery isn't just about the body; it's also about the mind. Taking time to rest and recover helps reduce stress, prevent burnout, and maintain a positive attitude on your fitness journey. Mental recovery is important for sustaining motivation and avoiding overtraining.

Types of Recovery

Recovery can be divided into two main types: active and passive. Both are important for overall well-being and should be incorporated into your routine.

1. Active Recovery

Active recovery involves participating in low-intensity activities that promote blood flow and aid in muscle repair without putting additional stress on the body. Examples include:

- Walking: Light walking can help improve circulation and reduce muscle stiffness.

- Yoga: Gentle yoga stretches and poses can improve flexibility and promote relaxation.

- Swimming: Low-intensity swimming or water aerobics provide a full-body workout without high pressure on the joints.

- Cycling: Easy cycling can help flush out lactic acid and lessen muscle soreness.

2. Passive Recovery

Passive recovery involves total rest and relaxation, allowing your body to heal and rejuvenate. Examples include:

- Sleeping: Getting adequate sleep is the most important form of passive recovery.
- Napping: Short naps can help recover your energy levels during the day.
- Massage: Professional or self-massage can lower muscle tension and promote relaxation.
- Hydrotherapy: Techniques such as hot baths, ice baths, or contrast baths (alternating hot and cold) can help in muscle recovery and reduce inflammation.

Techniques for Better Sleep

Sleep is a cornerstone of good recovery. It's during sleep that your body undergoes major repair and restoration processes. Here are some methods to improve the quality and duration of your sleep:

1. Establish a Sleep Routine

Creating a consistent sleep pattern helps regulate your body's internal clock, making it easier to fall asleep and wake up at the same time each day.

- Set a Bedtime: Choose a bedtime that allows you to get 7-9 hours of sleep each night and stick to it, even on weekends.

- Wake Up at the Same Time: Consistency in your wake-up time reinforces your sleep-wake routine.

2. Create a Sleep-Friendly Environment

Your sleep environment plays a significant part in the quality of your sleep. Here's how to improve your bedroom for rest:

- Keep It Cool: A cooler room temperature (around 60-67°F or 15-19°C) is helpful to better sleep.

- Darken the Room: Use blackout shades or an eye mask to block out light.
- Reduce Noise: Use earplugs or a white noise machine to drown out disturbing sounds.

- Comfortable Bedding: Invest in a good mattress and blankets that provide adequate support and comfort.

Limit Stimulants

Certain drugs can interfere with your ability to fall asleep and stay asleep.

- Avoid Caffeine: Limit caffeine intake, especially in the afternoon and evening.
- Limit Alcohol: While alcohol may make you feel sleepy, it can disrupt your sleep cycle and lower sleep quality.
- Reduce Nicotine: Nicotine is a stimulant that can make it difficult to fall asleep.

Day 13: Staying hydrated and how it affects metabolism

We can't say enough good things about how important water is to our health. On Day 13 of your two-week trip, we'll talk about staying hydrated and how important it is for your metabolism and health in general. Knowing why water is important and how to stay properly hydrated can make a big difference in your health and help you keep making the positive changes you've been working on.

Why water is important

About 60% of the human body is water, and it plays a role in almost every bodily process. Here are some important reasons why drinking water is good for your health and metabolism:

1. "Speeding Up Your Metabolism"

Water is a very important part of metabolism. It helps your body turn food into energy through a process called thermogenesis. Drinking water, especially cold water, can briefly boost your metabolism as your body works to warm it up to body temperature. Studies have shown that drinking 500 milliliters of water can improve metabolic rate by up to 30% for about an hour.

2. Aiding Digestion

Proper hydration is important for efficient digestion. Water helps dissolve nutrients and minerals from food, making them more available to the body. It also helps in the elimination of waste products, preventing constipation and promoting regular bowel movements.

3. Supporting Detoxification

Your kidneys rely on water to clear waste from the blood and excrete it through urine. Staying hydrated ensures that toxins are effectively removed from your body, reducing the load on your organs and improving overall health.

4. Regulating Body Temperature

Water helps control your body temperature through sweating and respiration. Proper hydration ensures that your body can efficiently manage heat, preventing overheating and keeping a stable internal environment.

5. Enhancing Physical Performance

Dehydration can impair physical function, causing fatigue, reduced stamina, and muscle cramps. Staying hydrated is important for maintaining energy levels, muscle function, and overall physical performance, especially during exercise.

6. Supporting Mental Function

Even mild dehydration can affect cognitive function, leading to impaired focus, memory, and mood. Ensuring adequate hydration benefits brain function and mental clarity.

Hydration Tips

Maintaining proper hydration requires a conscious effort to drink enough fluids throughout the day. Here are some useful tips to help you stay hydrated and support your metabolic health:

1. Drink Plenty of Water

The most simple way to stay hydrated is to drink water. Aim for at least eight 8-ounce glasses (about 2 liters) of water per day, though individual needs may vary based on factors like activity level, climate, and general health. Carry a reusable water bottle with you to make it easy to sip throughout the day.

2. Monitor Your Urine

A simple way to gauge your hydration status is by checking the color of your urine. Pale yellow urine typically indicates proper hydration, while dark yellow or amber urine suggests you need to drink more water.

3. Eat Water-Rich Foods

Incorporate foods with high water content into your diet to boost hydration. Fruits and vegetables like cucumbers, watermelon, oranges, strawberries, and lettuce are excellent choices that contribute to your daily fluid intake.

4. Start Your Day with Water

Kickstart your metabolism and hydrate your body by having a glass of water first thing in the morning. This practice helps replenish fluids lost during the night and sets a good tone for the day.

5. Flavor Your Water

If you find plain water unappealing, try adding natural tastes like lemon, lime, cucumber, or fresh mint. Infused water can make drinking more enjoyable and encourage you to drink more.

6. Hydrate Before, During, and After Exercise

Physical exercise increases your fluid needs. Drink water before your workout to start hydrated, sip water during exercise to replace fluids lost through sweat, and rehydrate afterward to aid healing.

7. Limit Diuretics

Beverages like coffee, tea, and alcohol have diuretic effects, meaning they can increase urine output and add to dehydration. While it's fine to enjoy these in moderation, balance them with extra water intake to keep hydration.

8. Use Hydration Apps

There are many apps available that can help track your water intake and tell you to drink regularly. Using technology can be an easy way to stay on top of your hydration goals.

Day 14: Reflecting on Progress and Planning Ahead

Congratulations! You've hit Day 14 of your transformative two-week journey. Today, we take time to reflect on your progress, celebrate your successes, and plan for the future. This final day is about analyzing the strides you've made, understanding what has worked well, and setting long-term goals to ensure that the positive changes you've implemented become lasting habits.

Evaluating Your Journey

Reflection is a powerful tool for mental growth. It helps you to assess your progress, recognize accomplishments, and find areas for improvement. Here's how to properly evaluate your two-week journey:

1. Review Your Goals

Look back at the goals you set at the beginning of this program. Have you met them? Consider both your successes and any places where you fell short. Reflect on why you achieved and what factors might have hindered your progress.

2. Assess Physical Changes

Evaluate any body changes you've noticed. Have you experienced weight loss, higher energy levels, improved digestion, or better sleep? Take note of how your body feels compared to two weeks ago.

3. Reflect on Mental and Emotional Changes

Beyond physical changes, consider your mental and emotional well-being. Have you felt more focused, less stressed, or more motivated? Reflect on any shifts in your thinking and mood.

4. Analyze Your Habits

Examine the habits you've formed over the past two weeks. Which new habits have you enjoyed and found sustainable? Are there any habits you fought to adopt? Understanding your preferences and challenges can help you refine your method moving forward.

5. Seek Feedback

If you've shared this journey with a friend, family member, or support group, seek their comments. Sometimes others can offer useful insights and perspectives that you might have overlooked.

Your two-week journey is just the beginning of a lifelong commitment to health and vitality. By reflecting on your success and setting thoughtful, long-term goals, you can continue to build on the positive changes you've made. Remember, true change is a continuous process that requires dedication, flexibility, and perseverance.

Embrace the lessons you've learned, enjoy your successes, and look forward to a future filled with energy, health, and well-being. Your journey doesn't end here—it's an ongoing adventure towards becoming the best version of yourself. Keep striving, stay committed, and enjoy the amazing benefits of a healthy, vibrant life. Here's to your continued success and health!

Conclusion

Congratulations on finishing your two-week journey to break free from cravings, boost your metabolism, and reclaim your vitality! Over the past two weeks, you have learned invaluable skills and information to transform your health and well-being.

As you move forward, it's important to sustain the momentum you've built and integrate these practices into your everyday life. This conclusion will guide you on keeping healthy habits and overcoming future challenges to ensure long-term success and vitality.

Maintaining Healthy Habits

Building and keeping healthy habits is the cornerstone of sustaining your newfound vitality. Here are some strategies to help you continue the good changes you've made:

1. Set Realistic Goals

After two weeks of intensive focus, it's important to set realistic, long-term goals that keep you motivated and on track. Reflect on your successes and identify areas where you can continue to grow. Goals should be defined, measurable, achievable, relevant, and time-bound (SMART). For example, you might try to exercise four times a week, prepare healthy meals at home five days a week, or gradually reduce your intake of processed sugars.

2. Create a Balanced Routine

A balanced routine includes various aspects of health, including nutrition, exercise, sleep, and stress management. Continue incorporating the ideas you've learned:

-Nutrition: Stick to balanced meals that include a range of macronutrients. Focus on whole foods, lean proteins, healthy fats, and plenty of fruits and veggies. Plan and prepare your meals to avoid hasty, unhealthy choices.

- Exercise: Maintain a regular exercise routine that includes a mix of cardio, strength training, and flexibility exercises. Aim for stability rather than perfection.

- Sleep: Prioritize quality sleep by following the sleep techniques mentioned earlier. A good night's sleep is important for recovery and overall health.

- Stress Management: Integrate stress-reducing activities into your daily routine, such as meditation, yoga, deep breathing exercises, or hobbies that bring you joy.

3. Monitor Your Progress

Regularly monitor your progress to stay accountable and inspired. Keeping a journal or using a tracking app can help you record your meals, workouts, sleep habits, and stress levels. Reflecting on your progress can highlight your achievements and identify areas needing improvement.

4.Stay Flexible and Adaptable

Life is unpredictable, and it's important to stay flexible and adaptable in your approach. There will be times when you can't stick to your routine due to travel, social events, or other responsibilities. Instead of feeling defeated, focus on making the best choices possible in each situation and get back on track as soon as possible.

5. Seek Support and Community

Surround yourself with supportive individuals who share your health and fitness goals. Whether it's friends, family, or an online group, having a support system can provide motivation, accountability, and encouragement. Consider joining exercise classes, support groups, or online forums to connect with like-minded people.

6. Celebrate Your Successes

Recognize and celebrate your successes, no matter how small they may seem. Celebrating your successes reinforces good behavior and keeps you motivated. Reward yourself with non-food-related treats, such as a relaxing spa day, new workout gear, or a fun trip.

Overcoming Future Challenges

While maintaining healthy habits is necessary, it's equally important to anticipate and overcome future challenges. Here are strategies to help you navigate typical obstacles:

1. Addressing Plateaus

It's normal to experience plateaus where progress seems to stall. Instead of getting frustrated, use this time to reassess your goals and habits. Consider making changes to your diet or exercise plan to reignite progress. Adding variety to your workouts or trying new healthy meals can also help break through plateaus.

2. Managing Cravings

Cravings can return even after breaking free from them. When cravings strike, use the techniques you've learned, such as identifying triggers, practicing mindful eating, and opting for healthier alternatives. Sometimes, giving yourself a small indulgence can prevent feelings of deprivation and help you stay on track.

3. Handling Social Situations

Social settings can pose challenges, especially when they involve food and drink. Plan ahead by eating a healthy meal or snack before going events, so you're not overly hungry. Offer to bring a healthy dish to share, and practice mindful eating during social events. Remember, it's okay to enjoy treats rarely, but moderation is key.

4. Dealing with Stress

Stress is an essential part of life and can impact your health and wellness goals. Continue practicing stress management methods, and don't hesitate to seek professional help if needed. Activities such as exercise, meditation, and spending time in nature can be particularly helpful in reducing stress.

5. Staying Motivated

Maintaining motivation over the long term can be difficult. Regularly revisit your goals and tell yourself why you started this journey. Visualize the good changes you've made and the benefits you've experienced. Setting new tasks and goals can also help keep your routine fresh and exciting.

6. Balancing Life and Health Goals

Finding a balance between your health goals and other aspects of life is important. Avoid an all-or-nothing mindset and accept flexibility. Life events, work duties, and personal responsibilities may sometimes take precedence, and that's okay. Focus on making the best choices possible in each scenario and maintaining a positive attitude.

Sustaining your energy beyond these two transformative weeks requires commitment, adaptability, and continuous effort. By maintaining healthy habits, anticipating challenges, and using the strategies described above, you can achieve long-term success and well-being. Remember, the path to optimal health is ongoing, and it's important to be patient and kind to yourself along the way.

Appendices

Embarking on a journey to reclaim your vitality involves not only understanding the theory behind your actions but also putting that information into practice through actionable and sustainable meal planning.

Below, you'll find a thorough guide to preparing wholesome meals that align with the goals set forth in this program. Each recipe is intended to balance your glucose levels, enhance your metabolism, and satiate your palate without leaving you feeling deprived.

Breakfast

1. Spinach and Feta Omelette:
   - Beat 3 eggs and pour them into a hot non-stick skillet.
   - Add a cup of fresh spinach and a sprinkle of feta cheese.
   - Cook until the eggs are set and serve with a slice of whole-grain toast.

2. Overnight Oats:
   - In a jar, mix ½ cup of rolled oats,
   - ¾ cup of almond milk,
   - a tablespoon of chia seeds,
   - and a dash of vanilla extract. Let sit overnight in the refrigerator. Top with fresh berries and a spoonful of Greek yogurt before serving.

Lunch

1. Quinoa Salad with Chickpeas and Veggies:

- Toss cooked rice with diced bell peppers, cucumbers,
- cherry tomatoes, and chickpeas.
- Add a sauce of olive oil, lemon juice, salt, and pepper. Garnish with fresh parsley.

2. Turkey and Avocado Wrap:

- Spread a whole-grain wrap with mashed avocado,
- add cuts of turkey breast, lettuce, tomato, and cucumber. Roll up the wrap tightly and cut in half.

Dinner

1. Grilled Salmon with Asparagus:
   - Season a salmon piece with lemon zest, salt, and pepper.
   - Grill alongside asparagus spears until the salmon is flaky and asparagus is soft. Serve with a side of quinoa or a mixed veggies salad.

2. Chicken Stir-Fry:
   - In a pan, stir-fry chunks of chicken breast with a mix of broccoli, bell peppers, and carrots.
   - Add a sauce of soy sauce, ginger, garlic, and a teaspoon of honey. Serve over brown rice or cauliflower rice for a lower carb choice.

Snacks

1. Hummus and Veggie Sticks:

    - Blend beans, tahini, olive oil, lemon juice, and garlic to make a smooth hummus. Serve with carrot sticks, cucumber pieces, and bell pepper strips.

2. Greek Yogurt and Nuts:

    - Mix a bowl of Greek yogurt with a handful of mixed nuts (almonds, walnuts, pistachios) and a sprinkle of cinnamon for a protein-rich lunch.